Günther W. Frank
Kombucha – Healthy beverage and natural remedy

Günther W. Frank

KOMBUCHA

Healthy beverage and natural remedy

Its correct preparation and use

PUBLISHING HOUSE ENNSTHALER STEYR

Disclaimer

This book is informational only and should neither be considered a medical advice nor a substitute for consultation with a duly licensed medical doctor or naturopath. Drinking Kombucha should not and must not replace any treatment prescribed by a doctor or a naturopath. Any attempt to diagnose or treat an illness should come under the direction of a qualified health professional before using any procedures where there is any question as to its appropriateness.

The author, the publisher and distributors are not responsible for any adverse effects or consequences resulting from the use of any of the suggestions, preparations, or procedures in this book.

www.ennsthaler.at

10th revised and updated edition 2018

ISBN 978-3-85068-337-1
Original title:
Günther W. Frank: Kombucha. Das Teepilz-Getränk

Translated into English by Miss Althea Tyndale
Translator of the updated edition: Helen Macfarlane

All rights reserved
Copyright 1991 by Ennsthaler Verlag, Steyr
Ennsthaler Gesellschaft m.b.H & Co KG, 4400 Steyr, Austria
Publisher: Ennsthaler Verlag
Cover picture: © GreenArt / Fotolia.com
Layout and Cover design: Thomas Traxl & Ennsthaler Verlag, Steyr
Printed by: Print Group, Szczecin

Contents

Foreword and Introduction

The tea mushroom kombucha, also known as SCOBY (Symbiotic Culture of Bacteria and Yeast), is an ancient folk medicine and household remedy. Over generations, the effects of kombucha have been coveted and cherished by many different nations, above all in East Asia. Many of our own elders, particularly from the then East Prussia, the Baltic countries and some parts of Silesia and Saxony, still remember how, as children, they would see their grandmother sitting in her warm corner, tending a mug of sweet tea with tea mushrooms floating in it. The tried, tested and treasured beverage was prepared for the whole family under her watchful eye.

Today, many people are turning to natural foodstuffs, remedies and stimulants. By activating the immune system and powers of self-healing, kombucha can support the regeneration and stabilization of health, fitness, activity and well-being. This fermented drink is not just for people with medical conditions, but, also acts as a foodstuff keeping the body in balance. Indeed, Kombucha is recommended by many traditional healers and doctors practicing naturopathic treatment.

Kombucha transforms tea into a healthy, nutritious detoxifying beverage

Communalities of yeasts and bacteria have been used by people all over the world, and applied for their well-being and the creation of health-promoting fermented drinks and foodstuffs since ancient times.

An ancient, pure member of these related symbioses of bacteria and yeasts is the tea-mushroom, kombucha. Although commonly known as the "kombucha mushroom", it is not a mushroom at all. It is a symbiotic culture of yeast and several different strains of bacteria grown on sweetened black or green tea. That is why the kombucha culture is also called SCOBY (symbiotic culture of bacteria and yeast).

The kombucha culture consists of a gelatinoid and tough mushroom-web membrane in the form of a flat disk. It looks like a white rubbery pancake. The culture is placed on or in the tea which is allowed to ferment for 8-14 days. It constantly multiplies through germinating. The fungal disk at first spreads over the entire surface of the tea and then thickens. When one treats the mushroom correctly, it thrives, germinates, and will accompany its owner for life.

A natural, tiny biochemical factory

During the fermentation and oxidation processes, kombucha affects diverse complicated reactions in the tea-setting, either one after the other or side by side (these are assimilation- and dissimulation-processes). The kombucha culture feeds on the sugar and, in exchange, produces other valuable substances which change into the drink: glucuron acid, glucuronic acid, acetic acid, lactic acid, vitamins, amino acids, antibiotic substances, and other products. The kombucha culture is, therefore, a real, tiny biochemical factory.

One drinks 0.10-0.25 liters (4-8 oz.) of the tea every day for detoxification of the body. It has a slightly sour to vinegary taste perhaps similar to a cider. The glucuronic acid is used by the liver to detoxify certain compounds and is considered by many to be the main beneficial ingredient of kombucha tea.

My kombucha journey

I received this mushroom years ago, myself. Since then, I have been much preoccupied with this ancient East Asian natural remedy, this fascinating little chemical factory that produces so many different substances.

I have made hundreds of gallons of Kombucha which I have drunk with my family; I have conducted my own experiments, as well as studying everything I could possibly lay my hands on, on the subject of Kombucha. I am particularly grateful to the specialists, professors, doctors, naturopaths, pharmacists, chemists, etc., who helped me to make the theoretical background accessible to the amateur. I am also grateful for the fruitful exchange of ideas with the many men and women who have allowed me to profit from their many experiences, and failures, too.

As I was working through the various references, scientific works and articles, I realized that the deeper one delves into any domain, be it biology, medicine, physics or philosophy, the more obvious it is that it's almost impossible to find a full explanation for everything. I accepted that statements such as "That's the way it is, and that's that!" don't always reflect the truth, but belong rather to the realm of conjecture.

Only charlatans are omniscient

The fact of the matter is, as the well-known physicist Professor Heinz Meier-Leibnitz put it in an article in WELT (World No. 295, of 17.12.88): "In every field, particularly in science, there is a tremendous amount that one simply does not know. 'We don't know' is a thoroughly scientific statement. Every scientist must not only know that, but also publicly admit it, and the public must accept it and neither expect nor demand omniscience. Only charlatans are omniscient and have an answer to everything. (...) It is very rare that something is thoroughly and accurately known and understood. Previous information often has to be corrected, or there are several bits of information of equal importance, but one cannot decide which one comes nearest to the truth."

And this is how Professor Ulrich Beck illustrated this fact in an essay in SPIEGEL (Mirror – No. 9/1988, pp. 202 – 201): "Whenever a motley bunch of experts is asked some question – for instance, 'Is formaldehyde poisonous?' – you'll get 15 different answers from let's say 5 scientists, all hedged about with 'yes-buts' and 'on the one hand – on the other hand' – if those asked are good; it they're not, you'll get two or three apparently definite answers."

As a consequence, I realized that I should regard the varying opinions emerging from the wide range of empirical experience and research work as being of value, even if I don't agree with them.

I don't like books which say "You must only do it like this. This is the only proper way to do it!" Counterarguments are withheld because they don't fit in with the author's own line of reasoning. When I then delve deeper and have a look at other sources, I perceive that these alleged facts are not at all as reliable as the author would have us believe.

I consider it matter of credibility and moral obligation that I should mention everything which can help the reader form an opinion, and also that I should not withhold anything which could be useful to those who think differently. Perhaps a book like this may present many readers with too much information. In that case, they might like to just cherry-pick the parts which seem most important to them.

It's your own responsibility
1. To form an opinion, there are two basic requirements:
2. Inform yourself to the full – seek and demand to know everything necessary. The fullest possible information must be sought and – that is, one must acquire adequate knowledge.
3. Exercise your own ability to think and judge - evidence must be assessed, discarded, evaluated according to one's own scale of values.

It's my job to make sure the reader is as well-informed as possible, so that he or she doesn't have to lend credence to every report and review. One has to be particularly cautious concerning statements by people who don't know anything about kombucha, or who only think they know something because they once happened to read a superficial and biased account in some leaflet or other, but who otherwise have never taken the slightest trouble to venture further and look up the references. Comments from such people sometimes remind me of the saying, "The less you know, the more certain you are."

Judge for yourself
If anyone should warn you against drinking kombucha or making the beverage yourself, I would recommend that you find out exactly who is offering this advice. Is this person competent to contribute to the Kombucha question? On what do they base their opinion?

What interests lie behind it? Binder and Wahler write (1988, p. 91): "Everything you can think of is proved by scientific studies these days." And Dr. Bruker says (1989; p. 7): "Objective and disinterested information has become a rarity in our times."

I have tried to write this book as I would wish a book to be: it must provide the fullest possible information and facts, without however forcing anything on the reader. I am not so presumptuous as to feel I should comment on every peculiar opinion; I let the various authors speak for themselves.

Let's take responsibility for our own health
Where there are alternatives, the choice of the right decision should be left to the reader. The decision may turn out to be different with each person, depending on how high one rates the advantages and disadvantages of any given point – and yet in relation to each person, their decision may be the right one. It's the same when you prepare Kombucha. There are many decisions possible, on many issues. What sort of sugar? How much sugar? How long should it be left to ferment? What kind of tea? But the reader must first of all have the facts, in order to arrive at the right choice. He has to know the pros and cons. Then he can compare and contrast, try out his own experiments, make his own mistakes – and in the end, reach his own conclusions.

Finding the truth through trial and error
Progress depends on the above-mentioned capacity to make mistakes, coupled with the ability to learn. The phrase "trial and error" aptly sums it up. That's why I don't ever want to relinquish either my capacity to make mistakes, or my ability to learn. This book reflects the present state of my knowledge. As for the future, I agree with what the composer Benjamin Britten says: "Learning is like rowing against the stream. As soon as you stop, you drift back again."

There are further questions I'd like to ask. There are further new experiences, information and results of experiments I'd like to evaluate. I'd like to continue improving this book about Kombucha and keep it permanently up to date.

If you ask me for my personal opinion concerning Kombucha, I'd say I'm absolutely convinced about the benefits it offers. When you've read so many reports and heard so much from the people concerned, you can't simply dismiss their faith in kombucha – based on personal experience – as humbug, just because everything doesn't happen to be analytically dissected. The reports from Russia alone, where research into Kombucha was carried on again after the war and sound, scientific investigations were carried out, elicit astonishment even from those skeptics.

Kombucha will reproduce itself with every batch

The good thing about the kombucha beverage is that it can be made at home with little money. As the culture continuously grows, you can start with a piece of the kombucha membrane and allow a health-promoting source of drink to ferment. The preparation is easy if you know how. Because the culture grows generously and is easily parted, all friends and acquaintances can soon benefit from it.

When you receive a kombucha culture you can cultivate it following the instructions in this book, and then pass on the resulting offspring to your friends, as a sign of friendship and mutual helpfulness. It its important, however, always to include complete information, preferably this book. You will only be able to produce a beverage that is palatable, wholesome and effective, if you use the right instructions.

Kombucha treats many diseases

Nobody knows exactly how many people in our world drink kombucha today. I can only imagine that the exuberant enthusiasm surrounding it will die down at some point and sensational reports will make way for more sobering perspectives: namely, that as we are being bombarded by environmental pollution from all sides, kombucha can help us do something for our health and well-being. It can also provide us with energy to survive our daily stresses without getting damaged. However, as exciting as it sounds, we should remain modest and not forget that kombucha is not cure-all Kombucha does not heal specific ailments. The body alone can heal itself and fight off an illness. The only thing a kombucha beverage can effectuate is to support the human organism, activate its own bodily immune system thus mobilising its powers of self-healing.

Kombucha is a special type of foodstuff, a biological, probiotic beverage full of living, strong microorganisms and dynamic force.

I have a dream

I hope to draw attention to the research work done on Kombucha (research work which began so promisingly in the twenties, but then sank into oblivion) not just to open discussion on the subject, but, also to revive it on a scientific basis and to support it through further studies.

The final secret of this "Miracle Mushroom", as it is referred to in many publications, is yet to be discovered and there is still a lot of research needed to make kombucha accessible to a far wider audience. Yet, can those healing effects, which so many people relate to us, be really attributed to it? We still have a lot to learn.

Perhaps there is someone out there (who has experienced many of the benefits of Kombucha themselves) who will donate the necessary financial means to further the research of kombucha so that this folk remedy will also be discovered by the world of school medicine. The research into this tea mushroom should be revived on a scientific level and secured through serious study. Those who refuse to accept this folk remedy, as there isn't any clinical studies for it, do not appear to understand that hundreds of studies into the pharmaceutical scandal surrounding "Thalidomide", "Vioxx" and many more could not be prevented.

> *Two things which prevent the progress of medicine:*
> *Authority and Systems.*
> Rudolf Virchow (1821–1902)

It only remains for me to wish you every success in preparing your kombucha beverage, and to hope that you will reap rich benefits from its use. May kombucha come to take the place it deserves in your household.

Part 1

What can kombucha do for you?

Does kombucha have a therapeutic effect?

A considerable corpus of experience has been accumulated concerning kombucha tea. Especially in Asiatic lands and in Russia, kombucha tea has been used for hundreds of years, with good results, as a natural remedy. Besides its use as a refreshing beverage, nearly every article also mentions its medicinal value. Innumerable illnesses are cited for which Kombucha tea is used and extolled. The range extends from the slightest ailment to the gravest illness.

"Hager's Handbuch für die pharmazeutische Praxis" (1973, p. 254-256) is completely accurate when it states under the heading "Combucha": "Application: In folk medicine, for practically all illnesses, as a diuretic in edema, particularly for arteriosclerosis, gout, under-activity of the intestines, and stones. As a refreshing beverage, and after a longer period of fermentation, as table vinegar."

However, it is precisely the application "for practically all illnesses" – something which is based on trust, tradition, recommendation or personal experience – that it queried by many adherents of scientific medicine.

Prejudices against the folk remedy
Those who advocate a purely scientific approach and who have learned to think in categories about cause and effect, usefulness and harmfulness, probably share the feelings of Dr. Siegwart Hermann (1929), who writes as follows about his first dealings with kombucha:

"About 15 years ago I received a 'fungus' from Poland, which was apparently identical with the so-called kombucha, and which was said to possess marvelous therapeutic properties.

Despite the highly praised mysterious powers, or precisely because of them, I took no particular interest in the miracle cure and let the culture die. I was prejudiced against 'folk medicine' at that time ..."

Hermann uses the expression "miracle cure", which was probably current at the time, so that to quote him correctly, I must use it too, even though I consider it to be detrimental as a practical assessment, as it puts kombucha on a level with charlatanism.

But let's return to Hermann. He doesn't stick to his initial skepticism. Instead of a full stop, he writes a comma and continues:

"..., only a comparative study of our medicine and folk medicine taught me otherwise. I saw that most of our useful remedies were discovered by the people, and only after hundreds of years of use were they added to the body of scientific medical lore. It is true that folk medicine is encumbered with countless errors and with a great deal of superstition, and that lacking a scientifically critical method it is only with uncommon difficulty that it can free itself of such things. However, hidden inside many folk recipes and remedies is something that is true and good. The folk doctors of all peoples, the shepherds and herdsmen, the herb women and the 'wise women' of Germanic folk medicine discovered most medicinal plants and noted their medicinal benefits. By investigating into what is known as kombucha, the disregard of folk medicine that I had at that time swung to the opposite extreme."

Antibiotic components

There are numerous scientific works on kombucha. They speak of its therapeutic effectiveness through the gluconic, glucuronic, lactic and acetic acids contained in it, as well as the essential vitamins it contains. As Russian research in particular has shown, many of the substances contained in it have antibiotic and detoxicating properties, and play a vital role in the biochemical processes in the human body. In contrast to many drugs and their unpleasant side-effects, the active substances in kombucha work on the system as a whole, and through their properties which are beneficial to the metabolism, they can restore the cell membranes to normal without any side-effects, and thus promote general well-being. This is very important, especially in our day, when we are exposed to so many controversial influences, be they in food (there are now around 3,000 permitted food additives), in drinking water, or in the environment. We are unable to defend ourselves against many of these often harmful influences. We can, however, help our bodies by maintaining or restoring a normal condition – well-being and health – through the correct supply of substances which have a positive effect on our health. Even if reservations against such concepts are still sometimes very great, and not everything has yet been scientifically researched, even then there are many practicing doctors who, with the aim of preventive medicine in mind, are turning to new food-physiology assessments of the substances which we feed into our system.

Numerous doctors and scientists have examined the effect of kombucha as used in folk medicine. Astonishing and scientifically sound reports have come from Russia in particular.

Of course you don't have to take the trouble to read all the reports. You can also form an opinion about kombucha along the lines of "The less you know, the more certain you are." But if you do take into account all the accumulated experience and scientific reports from all over the world, based on observations that reach back over centuries, then there is a chance of coming to your own independent evaluation of kombucha. When, in addition to this, I also take into account the various often almost unbelievable oral reports of kombucha users, and to be on the safe side delete a few as probably being exaggerated, I come to the conclusion that there must be something in the effectiveness attributed to the kombucha beverage which one cannot simply dismiss as humbug or charlatanism.

Strengthening of the resistance to disease

Many of the beneficial effects attributed to kombucha require further research. Other active effects, however, have been thoroughly verified by scientific research and by practical experience, e.g. regulation of the intestinal flora, strengthening of the cells, detoxification and purification, co-ordination of the metabolism, antibiotic effect, beneficial effect on the acid/alkali balance, strengthening of the resistance to disease.

I personally value kombucha as a highly effective foodstuff, a useful natural product, a biological, living fermented beverage. It is an effective additional foodstuff for all health-conscious people, one which contributes towards the regeneration and stabilization of health, fitness, activity and well-being, through the safe stimulation of the individual immune system.

Magic power or myth?

Kombucha has been surrounded by a kind of myth. You can see that from the different names given to it (also see part IX of this book): "Champignon de longue vie" (fungus for long living), "Zauberpilz" (magic mushroom), "Wunderpilz" (miracle mushroom). What might appear to be a miracle cure may occur because some person took the right nutrients at the right time, but there is no such thing as a magic bullet drink or pill for perfect health. It takes time and effort to return health where the body has deteriorated.

I would like to see millions of people experience an improvement in their state of health, and kombucha is a powerful weapon in anyone's arsenal.

Kombucha – a cure-all for everything?
However, there is a caveat. Kombucha has outstanding acids and nutrients to offer, but do not expect that it will allow you to continue an unhealthy lifestyle with impunity. You can't ignore nutrition, smoke, drink and abuse your body, then expect kombucha to cover for you. It doesn't work that way. Kombucha can certainly become a major player in the healthy household but don't expect it to raise anyone from the dead. It is not a miracle, it is a beverage from a natural, healthy process of fermentation.

Fermentation is the process of inducing a chemical change in a complex organic compound by the action of one or more enzymes, which are produced by microbes. This process has served mankind since the dawn of civilization and even in our age of technological wonders, some simple God-given ferments continue to serve human health far more effectively and economically than all the drugs and complex compounds in the arsenal of modern science.

Conclusion: Kombucha is an outstanding, health-giving. immune-boosting drink. Kombucha is not a cure all and you should not expect miracle cures even though a few "seeming" miracles will surely occur in individuals whose bodies will respond rapidly to a habit of fermenting and drinking kombucha.

Kombucha is not a magic potion. It is not a means of attaining immortality. It also does not give one a carte blanche to follow an unhealthy way of a life. It would be nonsensical to lead a life of excess, and then drink a bit of kombucha to even things out. Keep this in mind and kombucha can be used as a household remedy and foodstuff, as it certainly has properties which are beneficial to one's health. Kombucha can then be a means of regenerating and stabilizing the resistance needed to maintain and restore health, and of supplying it with what it needs to function optimally. Kombucha can then contribute to our well-being. In this way, kombucha can be recommended to everyone as a friend whose presence should be duly welcomed in every home.

The positive effects of kombucha on your health – A look at literature

In a bibliography drawn up by Prof. Eduard Stadelmann in 1961, there are 260 publications mentioned which deal with kombucha alone. A considerable number have been added to it, in the meantime. I shall try to give a cross-section of the publications which deal with the health aspects of the kombucha beverage. For reasons of space, I cannot mention anywhere near all of the articles.

He who knows how to listen, hears wisdom.
He who does not know how to listen, hears only noise.

(Chinese saying)

An extensive World-Literature
Bacinskaya had already established by 1914 that the beverage was effective in regulating the activity of the intestinal tract. The author recommended drinking a small glassful before each meal, and gradually increasing the amounts.

Professor S. Bazarewski wrote an article in 1915 in the "Correspondence of the Natural History Society of Riga", according to which a folk remedy bearing the name of "Brinum-Ssene" was widely known among the Latvian population of Livonia and Kurland in the Baltic provinces of Russia. Literally translated, it means "miracle fungus." Bazarewski writes that the Latvian people accredit it with "wonderful healing properties for many illnesses." Some of the Latvians whom Bazarewski questioned thought that it helped headaches, while others assured him "that it is useful for all illnesses."

Helps cure constipation
Prof. P. Lindner (1917/18) writes that the beverage is chiefly used as a means of regulating sluggish bowels. Lindner also mentions that

the culture itself can be used, as well as the actual liquid. Lindner also adds that he received further details about the healing properties of kombucha tea from Regional Postal Secretary Wagner of Berlin-Charlottenburg: "This beverage had been recommended to him years ago in Thorn as a remedy for hemorrhoids, and he had indeed been cured by taking it regularly."

Prof. Rudolf Kobert, Privy Councilor, (1917/18) recalls that an "infallible cure for rheumatism" was prepared using the kombucha culture.

Medicine cures three tenths,
diet cures seven tenths.

(From China)

Prof. Wilhelm Henneberg also writes that a beverage prepared by means of the kombucha culture, called tea kvass in Russia, is used everywhere there and is reputed to be "a means of combating all kinds of illnesses, especially constipation."

According to **Dr. Madaus** in "Biologische Heilkunst" (Biological Method of Healing – 1927), the kombucha culture and its metabolic products have an excellent effect on the regeneration of cell walls and it is therefore an excellent remedy for hardening of the arteries.

General improvement of one's overall condition
H. Waldeck (1927) relates how the chemist in Russian Poland on whom he was billeted in 1925 during the 1st world war, brewed him a "marvelous little drink" for his persistent constipation. The chemist confided to Waldeck that he never let this "secret Russian remedy" run out, "especially as it is supposed to be good for just about every kind of illness" and "because of its naturally produced acid, it can successfully combat geriatric complaints and thus contribute towards a prolongation of life."

Prof. Dr. Lakowitz (1928) confirms Waldeck's statement that digestive disturbances are quickly alleviated by the mushroom-tea. Strong headaches and nervous disturbances also are alleviated experientially. Lakowitz comes to the conclusion: "An extensive spreading of the mushroom-tea for the production of such Tee-Kwasses, as a remedy against digestive disturbances is desirable for all types of people".

The "**Weissen Fahne**" (White Flag, Journal on Interiorisation and Spiritualisation 1928) reports that "the refreshing taste of the tea beverage is generally pleasing, and the effect, as far as can be judged from the short time it was tested, is very good. The taste of the fermented tea is very pleasant, and is somewhat reminiscent of semi-sparkling wine or sweet cider. The tea takes effect for the most part very quickly, cleansing the blood and removing waste products, and apparently, so our correspondent writes, it also has an excellent effect on bad rashes of spots on the face. According to expert medical opinion, it also has an excellent effect on persistent headaches, rheumatic pains, gout, rheumatism, as well as other complaints of old age. The general effect of the kombucha beverage becomes obvious after only a few weeks by a general improvement in the overall state of health and by the improvement in mental and physical capacity, which can be attributed to the high vitamin and hormone effect of kombucha, something incidentally that is also emphasized by doctors. In addition, kombucha is excellent for stimulating the metabolism, similarly to vitamin R, thereby helping to remove waste products from the body, i.e. eliminating all sorts of substances which cause disease".
Note: According to present-day views it is assumed that the glucuronic acid binds the waste products to itself and is eliminated with the urine (glucuronide or "conjugated glucuronic acid").

Dr. Maxim Bing (1928) recommends the 'kombucha sponge' as a "very effective means of combatting hardening of the arteries, gout, and sluggishness of the bowels". By using good fresh cultures" a very favorable effect begins to take place, which in cases of hardening of the arteries expresses itself by a drop in blood pressure, a cessation of feelings of anxiety, irritability and aches and pains, headache, dizziness, etc. The sluggishness of the bowels and their concomitant symptoms can be likewise speedily improved. Particularly favorable results are obtained in cases of hardening of the kidneys and the capillary vessels of the brain, whereas hardening of the cardiac vessels is less favorably influenced."

Dr. Siegwart Hermann (1929) describes experiments with cats which had been poisoned with Vigantol (an anti-rickets Vitamin B-preparation). He noted a positive influence in their cholesterol level when the animals received kombucha extracts. This is interesting because in cases of human arteriosclerosis there is also a raised cholesterol level. Hermann's resume based on these experiments is: "The observations by doctors at the sickbed, as also with the animal experiments, showed that folk-wisdom quoted effects have been observed in general."

In my opinion, the good effects Kombucha has been observed to have on gout, rheumatism. arthritis, etc., can probably be explained by the fact that harmful substances deposited in the body, through conjugation with the glucuronic acid contained in the beverage, are rendered water-soluble and made capable of being passed through the kidneys and eliminated with the urine. By conjugation, a sort of bio-transformation, exogenous and endogenous substances are bound with glucuronic acid as glucuronides, which are also called "conjugated glucuronic acids."

Professor W. Wiechowski (1928), the then Principal of the Pharmacological Institute of the German University in Prague, devoted an interesting treatise to the kombucha question, entitled "What stance should a doctor take on the kombucha question?" To my mind, Wiechowski displays a remarkable attitude of medical knowledge towards kombucha: "As mentioned above, it is in no way inconsistent with the principles of scientific medicine to use a remedy, the effective nature of which experimental pharmacology is not yet in a position to investigate. On the contrary, we frequently see that remedies which have long been used in therapy have only been explained comparatively recently by experimental pharmacology with regard to the nature of their effectiveness. (...) As kombucha is completely harmless as a medicine, there is no reason to warn the populace against its use, which for the time being is to be regarded as dietary rather than therapeutic."

Being stupid isn't not knowing much, nor is it not wanting to know much. Being stupid is believing you know enough.
A. J. Daniel (American novelist, 1921-1982)

Pharmacologist **Wiechowski** became convinced that the indisputable success obtained by drinking kombucha was not based on suggestion but on a real therapeutic effect of the beverage on the human organism. Prof. Wiechowski became convinced about the indisputable success of kombucha through the experiments which had been carried out at Professor Jaksch's clinic for internal medicine in Prague.

Dr. L. Mollenda (1928) writes that the kombucha beverage proved itself effective especially in disorders of the digestive organs, whose function it completely normalized. In addition, the beverage proved itself effective in cases of gout, rheumatism, and various stages of arteriosclerosis. He writes among other things: "Even though the beverage is acid, it does not cause overacidity in the stomach; it noticeably eases and promotes digestion even of indigestible foods."

Dr. E. Arauner (1929) writes about various medical opinions and assessments and arrives at the following evaluation: "To sum up, one can say that the kombucha culture and the extract produced from it has proved itself to be an excellent prophylactic for diabetes, and in particular for geriatric complaints such as hardening of the arteries, high blood pressure with its consequences such as dizziness, gout, hemorrhoids, and is at least a pleasant laxative." Dr. Arauner says that the kombucha culture has been used for hundreds of years by the Asiatic people of his homeland on account of its surprising success as the most effective natural folk remedy for fatigue, lassitude, nervous tension, incipient signs of old age, hardening of the arteries, sluggishness of the bowels, gout and rheumatism, hemorrhoids, and diabetes.

Recommendable for mental stress
The then Director of the state-recognized Pharmaceutical Academy in Brunswick, **Hans Irion**, says in his "Lehrgang für Drogistenfachschulen" (Training Course for Pharmaceutical Technical Colleges – 1944, Vol. 2, p. 405): "Through drinking the beverage, which is called tea kvass, a noticeable improvement in the whole glandular system of the body and a stimulation of the metabolism takes place. Tea kvass is recommended as an excellent prophylactic for gout and rheumatism, furunculosis, hardening of the arteries, high blood pressure, nervous tension, sluggishness of the bowels and signs of old age. It is also highly recommended for those engaged in sport and strenuous intellectual activity. Through the stimulation of the body's metabolism, excessive obesity is prevented or eliminated. Microorganisms get into the body along with the beverage, and they transfer harmful deposits such as uric acid, cholesterin and others in an easily soluble form and so eliminate them. Dysentery bacteria re suppressed."

Detoxifying in every regard
The first account in book form on the subject of kombucha was published in 1954. The 54-page booklet is written in Russian. The author **G. F. Barbancik** summarizes the most important results obtained by the use of kombucha as a remedy, in particular those by Russian authors. He reports its successful use in tonsillitis, diseases of the inner organs, especially those causing inflammation, gastroenteritis as a result of inadequate acid production, inflammation of

the small and large intestines, dysentery, hardening of the arteries, high blood pressure, sclerosis, etc.

In a short chapter, "Some groundless rumors concerning kombucha", Barbancik emphasizes that, seen from a scientific and medical point of view, the possibility that kombucha might have a carcinogenic effect is entirely without foundation.

In 1964, in the magazine "Erfahrungsheilkunde" (Empirical Medicine), **GP Dr. Rudolf Sklenar** from Lich in Upper Hessen wrote about his method of diagnosis and his therapy successes. "An outstanding natural cure consists of drinking a fermented beverage called kombucha, which has a detoxifying effect in every respect and dissolves microorganisms as well as uric acid and cholesterol." Dr. Sklenar had developed a biological cancer therapy in which kombucha, besides other biological remedies such as Colibiogen, plays an important role in rehabilitating the intestinal flora.

Dr. Sklenar reports that he was able to treat successfully with the mushroom-tea: gout, rheum, arteriosclerosis, arthritis, dysbacteria, constipation, impotence, nonspecific draining, obesity, furunculosis, kidney stones, cholesterol, cancer and especially its early stages, etc.

The glucuronic acid
In 1961, in the magazine "Ärztliche Praxis" (Medical Practice), GP **Dr. Valentin Köhler** stimulates discussion of the therapeutic use of glucuronic acid under the title "Glucuronic acid gives cancer patients hope." Glucuronic acid is one of the products which are formed during the fermentation process of kombucha tea. Dr. Köhler reported encouraging results from the treatment of cancer patients with glucuronic acid. If the glucuronic acid is left to take effect for as long as possible, it leads to an increase in physical resistance and possibly also in interferon production. The detoxifying function of glucuronic acid goes along with an improvement in the general state of health and the oxidative metabolism.

Dr. Köhler also observed surprisingly successful results in the **treatment of sick trees**. Scientific experiments were undertaken by several institutions in an attempt to solve the problem of dying trees. In the book "Sofortheilung des Waldes" (Emergency Cure for Dying Woodlands), published by Hans Kaegelmann (1985), Drs. Valentin and Julian Köhler write about the life-protecting function of glucuronic acid in Nature. Cell-building processes are triggered off or accelerated by nutrient ions, trace ions and heavy metal ions. The capacity of glucuronic acid to enter into a bond with harmful substances, either produced by the organism itself or coming from outside, effects a protection for the plant cells. In this way, more than 200 substances can be rendered harmless, even those which are contained in acid and radioactive rain as well as sulfur dioxide, nitrite, ozone. According to Dr. Valentin Köhler's experiments, the protective action resulting from the glucuronic acid also protects the genetic system of the plant from growth disorders or promotes the restoration of the same during the course of further growth. Thus in experiments with glucuronic acid it was even possible to back-breed "hanging geraniums" (they grew upwards again) and weeping birches (they grew upright again) – genetic influence!

What is valid for plant cells can also apply to human cells. If the processes of breaking down and building up in the human metabolism are maintained at the optimum level through the supply of small doses of glucuronic acid which is contained in kombucha, then a connecting link is made between scientific data and a natural product which at the moment is still favored mainly by the lay world. Here is a possibility of helping a humanity that is more and more endangered by harmful substances in the environment. Through glucuronic acid the "disruptive products" in the human body are broken down into end products, eliminated and thereby rendered harmless. This detoxifying function of glucuronic acid helps the many-sided functioning of the cells. This then becomes apparent in many people by an increase in endogenic resistance to the harmful substances and environmental pollution bombarding us from every side, in a resuscitation of the damaged cells in the body, and in a restoration and consolidation of well-being.

Helpful bacteria for intestinal flora

The yeasts and bacteria in kombucha help activate intestinal bacteria. Without a doubt, the millions of living yeasts and bacteria and the macro-molecules completely regenerate the intestinal flora. The lactic acid bacteria ensure a friendly, symbiotic environment in our intestine. The symbiosis of the mutual uses does not only consist of the named bacteria taking a place in our intestines and holding off dangerous species ensuring the survival of its own survival, but they also contribute to the digestion and to many other enzymatic processes.

The brothers and sisters of the kombucha tea mushroom

Kombucha has many brothers and sisters around the globe. Similar cultures of yeasts and bacteria have been used since time immemorial for the production of health promoting fermented drinks and food stuffs by people for their general well-being the world over. We can already read in the Bible (Ruth 2:14) that the wealthy farmer Boaz invited the Moabite Ruth, who would later become his wife, whilst he was gleaning grain in his fields, "Come over here. Have some bread and dip it in the wine vinegar!" And she sat down with the harvesters. He offered her some roasted grain and she ate until she was sated and left some over. This biblical scene which took place in 1000 BC, not only gives us some insight into the then, for our standards, modest yet exemplary nutritional habits, but we can also see that already in olden times lactic acid beverages were prepared using microorganisms and served as an energy drink and refreshment during the hard harvesting period. These natural products boost the metabolism and purify and detoxify the system. They stabilize health and make the system more resistant.

Experiments with water kefir

Another, refreshing, traditional, bubbly drink, a little like champagne, is reputed to have health benefits, too. It is produced from a symbiotic culture which has been given many diverse names: Water Kefir, Japanese Sea Crystals, Tibi, California Bees, Graines vivantes. The whitish, transparent "gristly" clumps are cultivated in water and "fed" with a little sugar and some raisins or figs. Thus, the fermenting crystals cause an intensive fermentation and multiply themselves. I experimented with water kefir for a long time, carrying out many individual experiments. Water kefir is an interesting and attractive object. I came, however, to the conclusion that kombucha can be assessed as being more valuable, from the point of view of health, due to its different components.

Part 2

Now we start

Where to get kombucha

Can you buy ready-made kombucha products?

There are two ways you can obtain this precious tea mushroom beverage. The easy variant is to buy a ready-made kombucha drink. Many people do not have the time or the opportunity to make kombucha themselves. They need not do without kombucha, but can obtain the beverage, ready-made, in bottles. Ready-made kombucha products are manufactured by various firms. The bottles are sometimes delivered to health food and whole food shops, chemist's and so on, or can be obtained through them.

Kombucha starter culture

The second way is to brew your kombucha beverage yourself. The traditional method to get a starter culture is from a friend, since every kombucha culture (the "mother") produces new kombucha babies (offsprings).

On the other hand, pass your kombucha babies on to other people. It is a good custom to pass on the kombucha mushroom to your neighbors etc. as a sign of friendship and mutual helpfulness. To help is a token of friendship. If you have received any benefits from kombucha (and I am sure you will), you should feel the moral obligation to tell others about it. As the Chinese saying goes: "Mutual help makes even the poor rich."

When starting a new batch of kombucha, it is important to get some kombucha tea as well as the starter. The kombucha tea should constitute 10% of your new batch. Adding the kombucha tea establishes the proper pH level (pH refers to how acidic the liquid is) of the solution and kick starts the whole growing process by introducing a large number of the proper microorganisms into the solution right from the start. Only beneficial organisms can live in this solution; other organisms die. This is one of the characteristics of kombucha.

Will each batch of kombucha be a success?

When you work cleanly and abide by proven directions, then there is no hesitation in making the kombucha drink, as in many generations past. Whoever has the necessary knowledge can deal successfully with the tea-mushroom – just as one deals with other "open" foodstuffs in one's household. When abiding by proven instructions, one can produce an impeccable, tasty, wholesome and effective kombucha beverage. The mushroom will increase and accompany its owner lifelong and serve him or her well.

The kombucha mushroom protects itself

Whoever treats his mushroom culture according to proven rules with thought and carefulness, need not expect disturbances. In the Russian reports it is even mentioned that no special precautionary measures are needed because the mushroom protects itself against impurities. It has a number of protective features: the organic acids, the low alcoholic content, carbonic acid, the antibiotic products all these jointly block the development of all foreign microorganisms not belonging to the tea-mushroom organism.

One hears now and again of people who don't succeed in producing kombucha properly. Dr. Siegwart Hermann mentioned (1929) that "the fermentation process, as commonly practiced, often takes an undesirable course, and infections from other bacteria and molds occur, which are often not entirely harmless and which can lead to unwanted and sometimes not entirely safe products." He therefore recommends working in general with uncontaminated cultures.

The reason for lack of success when you do it yourself, nearly always lies in the fact that you can't obtain information about exactly how it should be done, and so a lot of mistakes get made. Often the only directions budding kombucha fans can get hold of is a couple of lines, and when the inevitable questions arise, the available handbooks often diverge from one another, so that nobody knows what is actually correct.

The fact that each person will be working under different conditions must also be taken into account, e.g. as regards the quality of the water, the composition of the air, the degree of warmth, etc., so that each individual person making kombucha must find out for themselves how they can best adapt the handicaps to suit their own circumstances. Even scientific articles frequently mention varying results. As the kombucha culture is a living organism and exposed to all kinds of influences, which often cannot possibly be changed, the finished beverage doesn't always have the same composition and taste. Added to this, you can't always reckon on an unvarying combination of the composite parts of the culture. Conditions for development and propagation will be more favorable now for this kind of yeast, now for that, now for the Bacterium xylinum. Furthermore, the size of the culture in relation to the amount of the nutrient solution beneath it, and the size and shape of the fermentation container will be of significance, particularly in so far as this latter limits the expansion of the surface area of the culture and affects the admission of air during the process of fermentation. (See Dinslage and Ludorff, 1927).

To brew kombucha successfully, I think it is important to know how the various process which sugar actually does to the liquid during fermentation, why oxygen is needed, and why it is best to use black tea, then I can judge for myself and decide whether I want to weigh one disadvantage or other against some advantage, or not. So this handbook not only provides the reader with practical directions, but also equips him with theoretical background knowledge.

One should have at least some idea of the biological, biochemical and physiological processes which occur within the kombucha culture as well as within the human body, so as to be able to produce both a tasty as well as an efficacious beverage.

Of course, problems can arise during the preparation of kombucha, just as they do with other foodstuffs. This is often put forward as a reason why one should not make the beverage oneself. The same argument could be used against making your own jam, your own pickles, your own potato salad or any other food product you can think of. If you don't do things the proper way, mold and other harmful things can affect any food product.

The care of the culture and the preparation of the beverage are admittedly not entirely simple. Nevertheless, I'm convinced that anyone who really wants to can handle the culture perfectly well, just as they can handle any other 'live' food product in their home.

The culture has a long life-expectancy and possesses the ability to regenerate itself very quickly. At least, it has been reported that the culture was already in use as a remedy 2000 years ago among the Chinese. If it didn't possess such vigor, it wouldn't have lasted for such a long period of time until now. The Chinese didn't have any laboratories in which to raise the culture; and handing it down from generation to generation for hundreds of years didn't happen under the sterile conditions of a lab, but under the usual domestic circumstances of a normal family. So there's a good chance that the culture will survive your treatment of it, too, that it will keep on propagating itself, and that it will last you a lifetime.

Dr. Sklenar (from Lich in Hessen, died 1987), whom we have to thank for preventing the kombucha culture from being forgotten after the second world war, used such cultures for over 30 years in his daily surgery and handed them out to patients. He tried out a great many things, and eventually arrived at his recipe using black tea and ordinary white sugar. It would be of help to many, whenever they go wrong, if they stuck to the tested recipe of this experienced doctor.

To be successful, I would urge you to study the directions carefully right through and follow them closely, keeping within the range of variability. There is a certain amount of room for play which leaves you free to do your own experiments, trials and make discoveries.

Kombucha is not a substitute for consultation with a doctor
The medical and health procedures in this book are based on the training, personal experience, and research of the author. Because there is always some risk involved, the author and publisher are not responsible for any adverse effects or consequences resulting from the use of any of the suggestions, preparations, or procedures in this book. The author makes no claims regarding benefits of kombucha.

This book is informational only and should neither be considered a medical advice nor a substitute for consultation with a duly licensed medical doctor or naturopath. Any attempt to diagnose or treat an illness should come under the direction of a qualified health professional before using any procedures where there is any question as to its appropriateness. Nevertheless, the author is always interested in hearing about your personal experiences.

Man can advise and help;
Nature alone can heal;
and only God Almighty,
in accordance with His promise,
can do away with Death forever.

Dr. P.G. Seeger

Working with microorganisms: Absolute cleanliness is essential

Anyone who becomes interested in kombucha will soon find themselves involved in one small corner of the broad field of microbiology. This calls for particular care, thought and cleanliness.

Cleanliness is especially required for the containers used in preparing and fermenting the beverage, the work surface, our clothes, and even our own bodies too.

Mollenda (1928) writes as follows, concerning the handling of the kombucha culture: "The greatest cleanliness is recommended when dealing with the culture, so that you must always wash your hands properly with soap before handling the culture."

As far handling the kombucha culture is concerned, I don't think sterilization to laboratory standards is necessary. What we can take over from microbiological practice, however, is the following:

1. Containers should be treated at the highest temperature possible. Glass jars and other utensils should be scalded before use with boiling water, or water as hot you can possibly get it. Of course, if you want to be absolutely thorough, you can sterilize them in steam by placing them in an oven heated to 200 °C (fill the drip-tray with water to generate steam) or in a pressure cooker which can reach high temperatures. Personally, however, I find that's going a bit too far for normal home use.
2. You should wash your hands thoroughly with soap and then rinse them with water as hot you can bear.
3. It is advisable to set apart specific utensils (such as ladles, glass jars, pans, etc.) which will not be used for any other purpose than that of preparing kombucha.
4. You should set aside a special time for preparing kombucha, during which you will have no other business to attend to. If this isn't possible, after each time you have been called away you must wash your hands again.

5. The culture should only be kept out of the fermentation container as long as is strictly necessary. When out of the fermentation container it should at least be placed in a covered glass or china container.

6. Even after starting the culture off, the fermentation container is to be kept in the very cleanest condition possible. Placing the fermentation container in the vicinity of mildew or mold (e.g. wet or dry rot in walls) or of potted plants is to be avoided, as spores can be transferred from these sources.

How to make kombucha – step by step

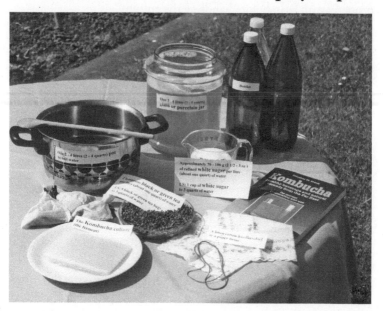

Ingredients

- The kombucha culture (the ferment) – Annotation: The culture is also called SCOBY (for symbiotic culture of bacteria and yeast)

- Approximately 70 grams (2½ oz) of refined white sugar per liter (about one quart) of water
- 2 teaspoons black or green tea per liter (about one quart) of water

Utensils and materials
- One 2 to 4 liters (2 to 4 quarts) pot to boil water
- One 2 to 4 liters (2 to 4 quarts) glass or porcelain jar
- A rubber band, a funnel, a sieve
- A linen/cotton handkerchief or a paper tissue
- Bottles for bottling the finished drink

In US standard measurements, it is mostly used this basic recipe: Make tea using 5 black or green tea bags, 1 cup of white sugar, and 3 quarts of water.

Procedure for the preparation of kombucha
It's best if you begin first with two liters (2 quarts). When your kombucha culture has grown big enough and has reproduced itself, you can produce larger quantities of the beverage.

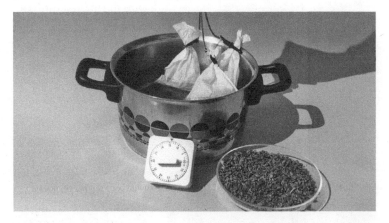

1 – Make tea in the ordinary way. Per liter (quart) of water, infuse 2 teaspoonfuls (about 5 g = 0.2 oz) of black or green tea in freshly boiled water. You may also use tea bags. Let the tea leaves "soak" for 15 minutes.

The best method is to use the following tea mixture: mix 1 part green tea (i.e. unfermented black tea) and 1 part "herbal tea", a herbal mixture described in the next chapter (yarrow, dandelion, nettle, clubmoss) at a ratio of 1:1.

Normally, you allow the green or black tea to brew for about 3 to 5 minutes. We brew the tea for kombucha longer so that more nitrogen passes into the liquid which the mushroom needs for its metabolism.

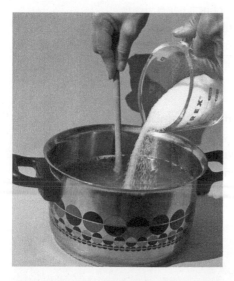

2 – Strain off the tea leaves through a sieve, or remove the tea bags from the water, as the case may be.

3 – Add about 70 grams (2½ oz) of white sugar per liter (quart) of water into the filtered infusion before it has cooled. Stir the tea so that the sugar dissolves totally. 1 tablespoon of sugar is about 20 grams (0.7 oz).

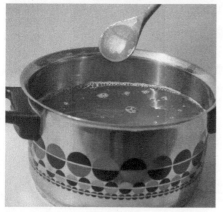

4 – Let the sugared tea cool down to a temperature not higher than 20-25 °Celsius = about 68-77 °Fahrenheit (lukewarm). The culture dies when it has been placed in a hot nutrient solution.

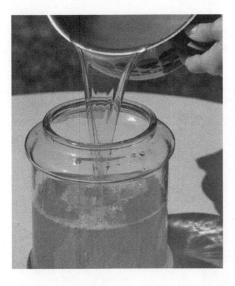

5 – When the tea has cooled to room temperature, pour the solution into a glass, china, glazed earthenware or stainless steel container. Glass is best.

Metal containers or other types than stainless steel are unsuitable and should never be used because the acids formed may react with the metal. You could also use a high-grade synthetic material of the polyolefin group, e.g. polyethylene (PE) or polypropylene. Wine or cider is also kept in containers made of this food-grade material. However, you should avoid containers made of polyvinylchloride (PVC) or polystyrene.

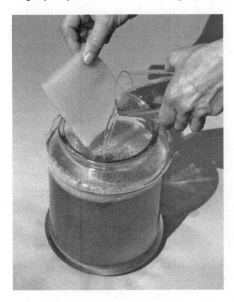

6 – When you prepare your first kombucha drink, **add the liquid that you got with the culture**. With all later batches, always keep enough kombucha drink to add about one tenth (10%) of the quantity to your new batch as a "starter liquid."

This is important to optimise the beginning of the fermentation process. The tea is simultaneously protected from damaging microorganisms. The acid environment prevents the development of any damaging bacteria.

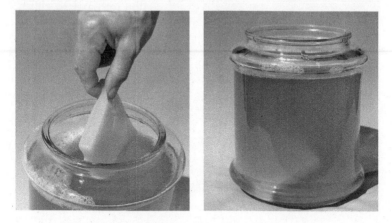

7 – Place the live kombucha culture in the liquid. Sometimes the culture floats on the surface, sometime it sinks to the bottom of the liquid. Both are OK. When the culture sinks to the bottom a new culture (a baby-culture) will begin to grow on the surface of the tea. For more details, see part 4 of this book. The kombucha culture needs some time to reproduce itself. It begins with a thin and filmy layer. The longer you leave it in peace, the thicker the new culture will grow.

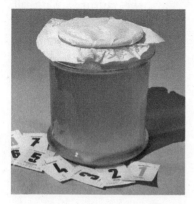

8 – Cover the mouth of the fermentation container with a tightly woven fabric, a tea towel, paper towel or similar light cloth to keep out fruit flies, dust, plant spores and other pollutants. Secure it with a large rubber band to ensure that fruit flies can't get in. The cloth must be porous enough

to allow air to circulate so the culture can breathe, but not so porous that tiny fruit flies can get in to lay their eggs.

9 – The fermentation should proceed for 8-14 days, depending on the temperature. The higher the room temperature, the faster the fermentation. The period of 8-14 days is given merely as a guide.

The kombucha culture needs a warm and quiet place and should on no account be moved. The temperature of the tea should not fall below 68 °F (= 20 °Celsius) and not rise above 86 °F (= 30 °Celsius). The ideal temperature is about 74-80 °F (= 23-27 °C). Light is not necessary. The culture also works in darkness. The culture may be damaged by exposure to bright sunlight. Half shade is better.

During the process of fermentation, the sugar is broken down by the yeast and converted into a gas (CO_2) and various organic acids and other compounds. It is the combination of these processes which gives the kombucha beverage its characteristic flavor.

If a slightly sweet drink is preferred, the fermentation has to be stopped earlier. For a dry or slightly acid flavor, it has to be continued longer.

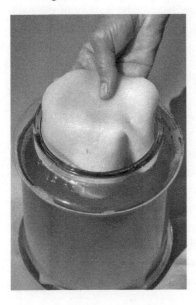

10 – When the tea has attained the right acid degree (pH 2,7-3,2), depending on individual taste, remove the culture with clean hands. From time to time, clean the culture under cold or lukewarm water. Fill the jar with fresh tea and add the culture. Respect the right temperature of the tea.

If you do not start a new batch immediately, place the culture temporarily in a covered glass or porcelain container.

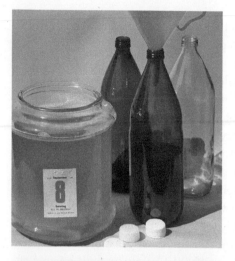

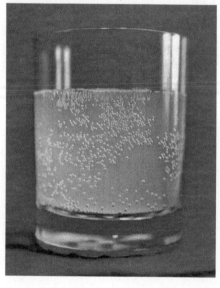

11 – Pour the beverage into bottles, which should be filled to the brim. Keep about one tenth (10%) as starter for the next batch. Possibly use a sieve to avoid fluff or film (harmless parts of the microorganisms).

Stopper the bottles securely.

12 – To find ultimate satisfaction in this drink it should be allowed to mature for a few days (at least 5 days), after having been bottled.

The activity of the bacterium is stopped because the bottling excludes the air, while the yeast continues to work. If the bottles are securely stoppered, the gas produced by the yeast's activities, is unable to escape. Thus an effervescent drink is produced. The drink has an agreeable taste. It is sparkling, slightly sour and refreshing. For this a few days in the bottles is usually sufficient; the kombucha beverage, however, will keep well for months. Do not worry: The yeast will stop the gas production at a certain point.

It is advisable to keep the beverage in a cool place.

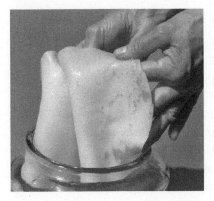

13 – After filling up the storage containers (the bottles) with the ready beverage, begin a new fermentation process. From time to time, wash the mushroom carefully under running cold or lukewarm water and put it back into the fermentation container. A new kombucha culture grows gradually over the surface of the liquid. Once it is ½ to 1 cm thick, you can remove it and use the original mushroom for the process. You can take the new mushroom and cut it in half with scissors so you have two half moons. Take one of these for the next preparation and give the other one to a friend...and so on. Leave the yeast sediment in the fermentation container, pouring it out every four to eight weeks and rinsing the container with hot water. If the beverage turns out to be too sour, remove the yeast sediment more often.

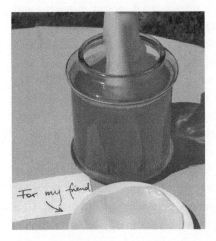

For my friend

14 – Start at step 1 again and make your own vitalizing drink which also lives! Here's to your success! When you start a new fermentation process, never forget to add to the new tea at least 10% of the liquid from a cultivation which has already fermented.

One normally drinks three glasses a day, one glass (0.1 liter/quart or more) on an empty stomach in the morning, the second glass after a meal in the course of the day, and the last glass a short time before going to bed.

45

Important point to be noted

Growing a new culture usually takes longer than the normal fermentation process. You should therefore separate the cultivation of a new kombucha-baby from the preparation of your beverage. This works as follows

Take two jars, the first for producing the beverage that you plan to drink and the second for growing a new kombucha baby. Half fill the second jar with the fermented beverage and pour in about the same amount of fresh tea (cooled!).

Add a small amount of the mushroom in the liquid of the second jar. You can simply cut off a small piece (about 3cm in diameter) of any mushroom using scissors. Or you can place the thin skin which has formed after 10-14 days, in this glass. When the second culture or thin skin sinks into the liquid, a third baby-culture forms on the surface.

Leave the second fermentation glass for growing a new kombucha baby alone for about 4 to 8 weeks. As with many wonders of nature, the new tea mushroom needs time to grow… so **be patient!**

In this way each culture will continue to propagate itself until it gradually begins to turn a dark brown color. When it is dark and dirty brown discard it and replace it with one of its offspring. Thus, this unique culture can provide you, your family and your friends with an ongoing supply of kombucha tea at very low cost.

Time and time again, I'm asked the same questions: "Why do you need so much sugar? And why do you have to let the tea brew for 15 minutes, when normally 5 minutes is enough at the most?" These subjects are dealt with in detail later on, so for the moment, simply and briefly:

The nutrient solution has to feed the microorganisms in the kombucha culture, not us. We must therefore prepare the nutrient solution according to the requirements of the yeasts principally (the bacteria feed in their turn partly on the nutrient solution itself). The microorganisms need the sugar in order to become activated. In nutrient solutions with a low concentration of sugar (carbohydrate), correspondingly fewer active substances are released. In lay terms, the sugar is "eaten" by the yeasts.

The tea infusion, on the other hand, serves as a source of nitrogen and promotes the growth of the microorganisms. A rather longer time than usual is recommended for brewing the tea for as much of this nitrogen as possible to pass into the nutrient solution, as well as mineral salts, and so on. The Russian research scientist Danielova (1959) even went so far as to boil the tea for 3 to 5 minutes, presumably for the same reason.

Part 3
The tea

What sort of tea to use

All the scientific and semi-scientific publications on kombucha that I've been able to get hold of up till now mention only "black tea" or "Russian tea" in general terms, expect for one Japanese article which reports that green tea (i.e. unfermented black tea) has also been successfully used.

Just from this alone you can see that it's not vitally necessary to use a specific sort of black tea. A fact which must also be taken into account is that the results can differ due to local differences in water quality, even when the same sort of tea is used. So, for example, in East Frisia where the water is allegedly of poor quality, one can only make a decent cup of tea with the "East Frisian Blend", which I find too strong. In many areas it's the water (which the tea connoisseur prefers to be soft) which is actually the problematical part of making tea.

From my own experience, I can report as follows: For a while I used Ceylon tea. The tea and consequently the kombucha beverage tasted strong and were very dark in color. From various references, my attention was drawn both to Bancha tea as well as to green tea, and I then used green tea for a while with good results. It is a pleasant, mild beverage. Since then, I only use green tea (green Darjeeling or Gunpowder), which produces a balanced, mild, clean tasting kombucha beverage with a good flavor and attractive appearance.

You can also use mate tea (yerba mate, Ilex paraguariensis), rooibos or redbush tea (scientific name Aspalathus linearis) or pu-erh tea (a variety of fermented Camellia sinensis).

Green tea

According to various sources, either green tea or Bancha tea is recommended, as is mild smooth tea from China or Japan. These teas are very suitable indeed from the point of view of neutrality and flavor. Green tea is produced mainly in China and Japan. It comes from the same plant as black tea and is distinguished from it principally by the way it is processed: it is not fermented.

Immediately after being plucked, the leaves are lightly steamed to inactivate the oxidizers. Oxidation of the tannins is thereby prevented and the chlorophyll preserved. After this, the leaves are rolled and dried. Fermentation has not taken place. The tannin content is hardly reduced at all.

Green tea gives a very light-colored, clear infusion with a stimulating, bitter taste. Green tea comes nearest to the natural flavor of tea. In general, the caffeine content is rather lower than in black tea.

Gunpowder Tea is one of the best-known varieties of green tea. The name refers to the appearance of the leaves, which are rolled into little pellets that look rather like shot. Other well-known varieties of green tea are Chun Mee, Hyson and Jasmine.

Bancha tea is a Japanese variety of green tea with an especially low caffeine content due to the leaves and stems of the Japanese tea-bush being harvested during the cold season of the year. The three-year-old tea leaves, which are the ones mostly used for this, are picked in winter, when the tea plant is resting and the caffeine content is at its lowest.

The caffeine content of **Kukicha tea** is even less than that of Bancha tea. With Kukicha, which is cultivated in eastern Asia, it is not the leaves which are used to make an infusion but the twigs and stems of the tea bushes, which are only picked after three or four years or more. This tea is also known by the name of "Three Year Tea." Bancha and Kukicha have a strong taste and are very easy on the stomach.

Midway between black tea and green tea is Oolong tea, which comes from Taiwan (Formosa). Oolong tea is semi-fermented, and regarding its taste and to appearance, lies midway between black and green tea. The tea retains a particularly strong flavor because the fermentation is broken off early on.

The special value of green tea for one's health
In the beginning, tea was 'green'. In all matters concerning the history of tea, one thing is certain: for thousands of years, tea was drunk exclusively in its 'green' state, that is, unfermented. The medicinal effects of tea described in older Chinese and Japanese literature always refer to unfermented green tea.

The Chinese drank tea first of all for health reasons. It was regarded as a medicine, and was described in the earliest Chinese books on medicine. In Europe, too, tea first appeared in the apothecary's shop. Later on, once people had acquired a taste for it, it was classed as a luxury item.

Particularly in the 20th century, painstaking chemical and physiological research revealed that green tea is marvelous medicine. Victims of the atom bomb explosion in Japan drank a lot of green tea, and thereby saved their lives.

Teidzi Ugai and Antsi Hayashi of Kyoto University write that green tea is effective against Strontium 90, one of the most harmful radioactive isotopes therefore against cancer and leukemia.

The vitamin C in fresh tea leaves is said to be four times higher than in lemon or orange juice. As for the vitamin B content, no other plant comes anywhere near green tea. (The source of this piece of information cannot be ascertained.)

Green tea is said to make the blood vessel walls more elastic, prevent cerebral hemorrhage and heart attacks, and lower abnormal pressure in the arteries.

Dr. Berieva, a Turkmen specialist, did some research into infectious diseases, and it was noticed that in Turkmenistan, where people drink a lot of tea, dysentery does not occur. Experiments in the Botikin Hospital, Moscow, established that tea is preferable to antibiotics in the treatment of dysentery. In contrast to antibiotics, tea is completely harmless. Green tea seems to work best against microbes.

Dr. Berieva apparently prescribed green tea for patients suffering from dysentery and typhoid fever. Even in the worst cases, the dysentery bacteria disappeared in only 2 or 3 days after treatment began. Complete recovery occurred between the 8th and the 10th day. The usual treatment lasts for weeks. In the check-up that followed six months later, not a single patient turned out to be a carrier.

It has been reported that green tea has been used successfully in cases of hemorrhaging in the gastric canal and intestinal tract and for cerebral hemorrhage, as well as for brittleness of the capillaries due to old age. It is reputed to be an excellent remedy for bladder stones, gall stones and kidney stones. Vitamins B2, P and K, which are to be found in green tea, make the skin feel elastic and fresh, strengthen the capillary walls, and prevent subcutaneous bruising which causes the build-up of blue blood vessels and blotches.

However, it was an article in GEO magazine (November 1987) which convinced me most about the health value of green tea, and I quote it here verbatim with the kind permission of the publisher (Gruner + Jahr AG & Co, Hamburg).

Cancer research – Green tea inhibits the growth of tumors

Unfermented green tea is not only a stimulating pleasant tasting beverage, but also prevents the growth of cancer tumors. Hirota Fujiki and his colleagues at the National Cancer Research Institute in Tokyo have just recently come to this conclusion. Statistical surveys by the Japanese Public Health Department gave medics an important clue. According to these studies, fewer people died of cancer in the Prefecture of Shizuoka, where green tea is grown and drunk in large quantities, than in other areas of Japan.

Fujiki and his colleagues suspected that the tannins contained in green tea function as 'cancer-stoppers'. To prove their theory, they isolated the principal element of tannin from the tea leaves, epigallocatechingallate (EGCG).

The medics tested the effect of this substance by one of the standard methods commonly used in cancer research – they treated the dorsal skin of mice with a chemical which changed the normal cells into dormant cancer cells. Then they divided the mice into two groups. They gave a substance which encourages the growth of tumors – something that "promotes the growth of tumors" as the doctor would say – to the animals in the first group, at intervals of half a week each. They gave the same cancer-promoting substance at the same intervals of time to the mice in the second group as well, but in addition they gave each of these a dose of the presumed cancer-stopper EGCG.

25 weeks later the Fujiki team found that 53% of the mice which had been treated solely with the cancer-promoting substance had developed cancer growths. On the other hand, a mere 13% of the mice which had been treated with EGCG as well had developed tumors.

The Japanese cancer research scientists explain the effect of EGCG thus: The tumor-promoter normally settles on a specific 'receiver' on the upper surface of a mouse sell and re-programs it to become a tumor cell. But this is exactly what EGCG seems to prevent – it alters the receiver in such a way that the tumor-promoter can no longer 'dock' into it. Because of this, the mouse cell stays protected from attack by the harmful substance, and cannot develop into a tumor cell.

On the basis of the results of their experiments with mice, the Japanese doctors assume that EGCG from green tea could also prevent cancer growths in humans, particularly cancer of the esophagus, stomach and bowel. So Japanese tea-lovers are on to a good thing; at any rate, they're absorbing about a gram of EGCG daily through drinking green tea. Western tea drinkers, however, drink mostly black tea, which as a result of fermentation contains only minimal amounts of EGCG. So presumably the best thing to do in future would be to change over to green tea.

Caffeine content in kombucha

Green and black tea differentiate themselves through their caffeine content. Though, what we know as white tea, a slightly fermented tea, has a relatively high caffeine content in comparison to green and black tea.

The caffeine in black and green tea is not or very minimally reduced, thus it is necessary to take care with children and pregnant women (e.g. with sleep problems). In this case, black tea should be avoided and tea low in caffeine (e. g. Bancha) or herbal tea used.

Caffeine is a purine-alkaloid and a stimulating component of tea and other drinks. It is one of the oldest stimulants. It dilates the vessels and stimulates breathing and circulatory centers. Caffeine in black and green tea works differently to that in coffee although both "caffeine sorts" are chemically identical. The reason for these different effects is that whilst brewing black or green tea, **tanning agents** are released from the leaves into the water. These special bitter compounds delay the effect of the tea. These are not present in coffee. This explains why coffee acts as a faster and stronger stimulant, whereas, the effects of tea start working much later, but, therefore last longer.

When you pour hot water on tea, the caffeine, mineral nutrients and vitamins are released from the leaves first. After about a minute, practically all the caffeine is already in the water. The tanning agents which "save" the effects of the caffeine, so to speak, are released considerably slower from the tea leaves.

Would you like to use decaffeinated black or green tea?

You can use decaffeinated tea for your kombucha. You can, however, decaffeinate it yourself by brewing your tea for thirty seconds to one minute at the most. In this time the caffeine is released into the water. You can use this first tea infusion as a stimulating, caffeinated beverage or simply tip it out. Now, make a second tea infusion with the same tea leaves. Let this brew for about five minutes (for kombucha fifteen minutes). You then have made a tea with all the tea nutrients, antioxidants etc. but with as good as no caffeine.

A few tips about making tea

If the water is too hot, it makes green tea bitter. This is why tea connoisseurs only let the water boil for a short period of time and then cool to 80 to 90 degrees celsius. One rule of thumb is that the temperature of boiling water drops to 90 degrees celsius after 3 to 4 minutes and 80 degrees celsius after 5 minutes.

If you strain the brewed tea through a sieve with a normal mesh, little bits of tea get left behind in the liquid. Particularly with broken tea, a lot of tiny little pieces of the broken leaves slip through the mesh. There are various things that can be done to avoid this:

1. You can use teabags. Teabags have the disadvantage, however, of not being able to release so many substances as loose tea leaves can. Added to this, they are only available in a limited number of varieties. If you want to use your own blend of teas, I would suggest the following methods:
2. When the tea has stood long enough, it can be poured through a coffee filter paper. Or you could line a wide mesh sieve with a sheet of household paper towel, and strain the tea in this way.
3. Tea filters are another practical solution for saving preparation time. There are other methods of filtering tea available from various firms. The easiest and fastest way to prepare loose tea is with paper tea filters. Tea can be prepared quickly and easily by these methods, which involve the use of a holder and disposable filter bags made of special paper. The tea can be infused for the exact amount of time required. The remains don't get stuck in the pot, but can be consigned in one simple movement to the dustbin or the compost heap.

How can you make large quantities of kombucha tea?
When I began to produce larger batches for my family I bought two large stainless pots of 14 liters (15 quarts). However, it is time-consuming and expensive to boil, for instance, 28 liters (30 quarts) of tea. This brought me to this idea: To avoid boiling such large quan-

tities of tea, make a **tea concentrate** and dilute it with normal tap water. For instance, if you want to get 14 liters (4 gallons) of tea just boil 3 liters (1 gallon) of water but use the tea quantity for 14 liters (4 gallons) tea. Thus you get a tea concentrate. Fill it up with 11 liters (3 gallons) of tap water. So you get 14 liters (4 gallons) of tea as nutrition liquid for your kombucha beverage. If you have good, clean water, this method works perfectly. I have tried it.

Herbal teas

As a basic principle, black or green tea is recommended. The reason for this will be discussed in the next chapter. In spite of the advantages of black tea as a nutrient solution, there are plenty of people who use herbal teas to make kombucha with, either because black tea doesn't agree with them, or because, in addition to the effect of the kombucha culture, they want to bring in the therapeutic value of the herbs as well, or for whatever other reason.

Mollenda mentioned this possibility in 1928, even though he considered black tea to be the best nutrient solution. He writes: "From experiments which have been made, it has been established that kombucha thrives best with sugar in an infusion of sweetened Russian tea. (...) The culture can also be raised on any other decoction containing nitrogen, such as lime flower tea or strawberry leaf tea."

Prof. Henneberg (1926) made "good, fragrant beverages" using strawberry leaves, raspberry leaves, blackthorn and lime flowers. As a general rule, he mentions 5g of tea to 1 liter of water.

If you don't want to use black tea, you can use ready-made commercially available herbal teas, such as those for liver, nerves, or digestive tract, and you can use various mixtures of herbs, e.g. nettle with blackberry leaves, coltsfoot, plantain, hawthorn, birch leaves, strawberry leaves, lime flowers. For herbal teas, you need two or three teaspoonful per liter.

The medicinal herbs used in preparing teas for the stomach, bile and liver, however, can make the metabolic processes and formation of new cultures difficult, due to the high amount of bitter oils contained in them. Wormwood, sweet calamus, yellow gentian root, centaury, seeds of the milk thistle and masterwort belong to this class of herbs.

Rosehip and fruit tea are also very suitable, and yield an attractive looking and pleasant tasting tea which children enjoy, too. I have noticed, however, that the culture membrane doesn't grow as much when using rosehip tea as when using varieties of black tea.

Sorts of tea should be used which contain too many volatile oils (e.g. sage, peppermint, camomile, St.-John's-Wort), because such tea blends can, in the long run, alter the active substances in the kombucha culture. As a guideline, I have drawn up a list which can be found at the end of this chapter.

Of course, you can make up your own mixtures of various herbal teas. I tried out the following recipe on the recommendation of the Heilbronn pharmacist, Herr Norbert Harmuth, and I can thoroughly recommend this blend, if you don't want to use black tea:

yarrow 40 grams
dandelion 30 grams
nettle 15 grams
club-moss 15 grams.

This blend makes a very pleasant tasting beverage. You could get this herbal blend made up for you by the pharmacist or at a shop specializing in herbs.

Pastor Hermann-Josef Weidinger writes in the "Ringelblume" (Marigold) magazine (No. 4/1988) that he has had good results using the following tea blend, mixing the respective herbs in equal parts: yarrow, chickweed, nettle, oregano, dandelion leaves and woodruff.

He recommends a further tea blend, likewise mixed in equal parts: bilberry leaves, raspberry leaves, blackberry leaves and blackcurrant leaves.

You could make up other tea blends according to your own taste, e.g. equal parts of rosehips, nettle leaves and green tea (or green maté tea).

At any rate, it is always best to add to your own blend at least a portion of black tea or green tea, as this makes the best nutrient solution for the kombucha culture.

The tea can also be left to infuse for much longer. I recently heard someone say that the plant parts of herbal teas should only be filtered off after one hour.

What are the disadvantages of herbal tea compared with black tea?

In the countries where kombucha originates, the original recipe is nearly always made with an infusion of black tea. The kombucha culture isn't actually dependent on this substratum for its activity and growth, but experiments have nevertheless demonstrated that black tea produces the highest concentration of lactic and gluconic acid. Apart from its particular taste and specific medicinal effect, tea is important as a source of mineral nutriments for the culture. And in this respect, black tea seems to provide the best conditions.

Bing (1928) considers the purine content of black tea to be the characteristic element of the nutrient medium. He attributes the particular suitability of black tea to the fact that, of the semi-luxury beverages, it is this tea which has the highest purine content, viz. 2.108 – 4.108 % of the dry weight including caffeine. In the plant and animal kingdom, purine is found in great amounts as physiologically important combinations, such as uric acid, building blocks of the nucleonic acids (guanine, adenine) and xanthine alkaloids (caffeine, theophylline and theobromine). Bing describes the kombucha culture as a community of living things which are particularly adapted to a nutrient milieu and need this abundance of purine to maintain their own metabolism. Bing thus explains the breakdown of purine in the human metabolism – and so of uric acid as well – through drinking kombucha.

According to Bing, the tannin content of tea also has a part to play in the formation of zooglea (skin on the surface of nutrient solution). By choosing a certain tannin, he says, you can get a crinkled up zooglea formation that looks like tripe instead of the usual smooth surface.

In 1929, Bing writes that the kombucha maker often "commits the sin" of using elderflower tea, chamomile tea and other herbal decoctions instead of good Russian or Chinese tea for the nutrient solution, which alone contains the necessary purine. He considers that it "goes without saying that under such circumstances the desired process of fermentation cannot take place and the effects fail to materialize."

Dr. Jürgen Reiss (1987) followed the formation of ethanol (ethyl alcohol), lactic acid, gluconic acid and acetic acid, as well as the breakdown of glucose (dextrose), by means of photometric enzyme tests. It was apparent from these experiments too, that the kombucha culture forms the highest concentration of lactic and gluconic acid as well as ethanol when the nutrient solution is black tea. When Reiss's results are compared, one comes to the conclusion that black tea is undoubtedly the best nutrient solution.

Biochemical changes of other substrata through the action of the kombucha culture after an incubation period of 14 days (Amounts given are % of grams per liter)

Substratum	Lactic acid	Gluconic acid	Acetic acid	Ethanol
Black tea	2.94	2.52	0.08	1.07
Lime flower tea	0.07	0.06	0.30	0.04
Peppermint tea	0.14	0.04	0.01	0.005
Coca-Cola	0.07	0.46	0.01	0.15
Beer	1.43	0.04	0.56	not measured

(Source: Reiss, J., Der Teepilz und seine Stoffwechselprodukte – The kombucha culture and its metabolic products – Deutsche Lebensmittel-Rundschau 83, 286 – 290, 1987.)

Despite the above results, it will still not be clear to some people why black tea should be better. I will therefore try to explain the reasons:

1. Many herbal teas contain more volatile oils and greater amounts of phenol than black tea. These constituents have a bactericidal effect (i.e. they destroy bacteria) or a bacteriostatic effect (i.e. they inhibit bacteria), and can affect the bacterial components of the kombucha culture. The volatile oils accumulate in the upper part of the fermentation fluid. That's where the kombucha culture floats, or, when it sinks down a bit, where a new culture forms. So the volatile oils can work directly on the kombucha culture. They can change it in the long run, in that they suppress the development of the less resistant constituents in the membrane of the culture.

2. Herbal teas contain more germinal spores than black tea. Through the heating process during the production of black tea and through the fermentation, the germinal spores present in black tea are correspondingly damaged and decimated. Herbal teas, on the other hand, contain a great many germinal spores, particularly where they include herbs which grow very near the ground. They contain a great many soil spores which then germinate in the warm nutrient solution. The natural habitat for the overwhelming majority of microorganisms is soil. One gram of good topsoil is home to about a billion microorganisms. In other words: a thimbleful of topsoil contains for its size proportionately as many microbes as there are people on our planet (Dittrich, 1975).

These microorganisms do get into the air by way of the wind, but they are to be found in far fewer quantities on the leaves of black tea, which are harvested from bushes that grow to a height of 1 to 1.5 meters, than on plants which grow near the ground. You might raise the objection: "But these germinal spores will surely be killed off when boiling water is poured into the herbal tea!" Yes, that's partly true. Most bacteria and germs are destroyed at boiling point, but many only after prolonged boiling. And even then there are permanent forms, the spores of which are not destroyed by boiling. If you suspect that such spores are present in anything you want to preserve, it must be heated to over 100 °C, e.g. in a pressure cooker, which can reach more than atmospheric pressure. It this isn't possible, then you must boil it for hours on end, or boil it repeatedly. If any remaining spores have germinated during cooling, then the resulting schizomycetes will be destroyed at the second or third boiling (see Schmeil-Seybold, 1940, p. 378). Something similar happens during pasteurization – that is, repeated heating, but only at 60-70 °C.

To sum up, we can say that black tea is neutral. The lower content in germinal spores is beneficial to the fermentation process. Why shouldn't one use it then? Indeed, scientific experiments have demonstrated that black tea breaks down cholesterol and other fats in the blood and the body. An investigation of this kind was undertaken recently in Finland, in March 1987.

The more you exercise your judgment,
the less prejudiced you'll be ....
Frank Wedekind

Conversion US-measures into the metric system

1 gram (g) is equal to	0.035 ounces
100 grams is equal to	3½ ounces
1 ounce is equal to	28.35 grams
1 pound (16 ounces) is equal to	0.4536 kilogram
1 liter is equal to	1.057 quarts or 35 ounces
1 liquid quart is equal to	0.9463 liter
1 gallon (4 quarts) is equal to	3.7853 liter

1 cup is equal to 8 ounces or 250 ml or 226,8 grams
5 g black tea is 0.18 ounces (about 2 teaspoons full).

Percentage of volatile oils in commonly used medicinal herbs

(Drawn up by Günther Frank, from Fischer, "Heilkräuter und Arzneipflanzen" – Medicinal Herbs and Plants.)

Medicinal herb	Volatile oil content as %
Agrimony (liverwort)	c. 0.2
Angelica, true	0.015 – 0.1
Angelica, wild	0.6
Aniseed	--
Apple peel	--
Arnica	--
Bearberry	0.01
Birch	traces
Blackberry, leaves	traces
Blackberry, fruit	--

Blackcurrant, leaves	traces
Borage	traces
Calamus (sweet flag)	1.5 – 3.9
Camomile, common	0.5 – 1.5
Camomile, Roman	0.7 – 2.4
Caraway, common, fruit	3 – 7
Cat's-foot (chaste weed, spring cassidony)	--
Centaury	traces
Cherry stems	--
Chervil, herb	c. 0.9
Chicory, wild, root	traces
Chicory, wild, herb/flowers	--
Club-moss	--
Coltsfoot	traces
Comfrey	--
Cowslip, flowers	--
Cowslip, root	0.1 – 0.25
Cumin, fruit	2.3 – 5
Daisy	traces
Dandelion	traces
Deadnettle, white	0.5
Dill	2.5 – 4
Elder, flowers	0.025
Elder, berries	traces
Eyebright	0.15 – 0.17
Fennel, seed	2 – 6
Fennel, herb	traces
Golden Rod (Aaron's Rod)	traces
Ground Ivy	0.3 – 0.6
Hawthorn (Whitethorn)	--
Hibiscus, flowers	--
Hibiscus, leaves	c. 0.02
Horsetail (Equisetum)	--
Knotgrass	traces
Lady's-mantle (Alchemilla)	--

Lavender, fresh flowers	0.5 – 1.0
Lavender, dried flowers	1 – 3
Lemon Balm (Melissa)	0.05 – 0.33
Lime flowers	0.04 – 0.1
Lovage, herb	0.9 – 1.7
Mallow	--
Marigold (Calendula)	0.02
Marjoram	0.3 – 0.9
Milfoil (Yarrow, Pellitory, Bloodwort), herb	0.4 – 1.4
Milfoil, flowers	up to 0.5
Mint (crisped/curled)	up to 1.25
Mistletoe	--
Mugwort (Motherwort, Artemisia vulgaris)	0.026 – 0.2
Mullein	traces
Nettle	--
Oats	--
Oregano	0.15 – 0.4
Peppermint	up to 1.25
Pimpernel	--
Plantain, greater	--
Plantain, Ribwort	--
Raspberry, leaves	--
Restharrow	traces
Rose, common, hips	traces
Rosemary	1 – 2
Rowan	traces
Rue	0.1 – 0.7
Rue, meadow (galega)	--
Sage (Salvia)	1 – 2.5
St.-John's-Wort	0.05 – 0.9
Silver-weed (Wild Tansy, Potentilla anserina)	--
Shepherd's Purse	traces
Speedwell, common	traces
Strawberry, herb	traces
Tarragon, fresh herb	0.1 – 0.45

Tarragon, dried herb	0.25 – 0.8
Thyme, common garden	up to 1.7
Thyme, wild/creeping	0.15 – 1.0
Valerian	--
Wormwood (Absinth)	0.25 – 1.32

Part 4

The fermentation process

Starting off the kombucha culture in the fermentation container

Hot tea kills the kombucha culture. Wait, therefore, until the tea has cooled down to room temperature (20-25° Celsius = 68-77° Fahrenheit). It's not very easy to estimate the right temperature with your hand. It's best to buy a bath thermometer for this purpose, which should then be used only for preparing kombucha.

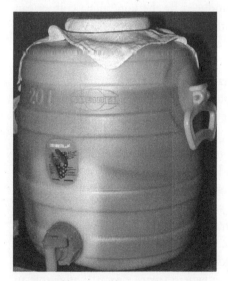

A container like it is used by wine-growers. It is made of food grade polyethylene (PE).

When the tea reaches the right temperature, pour it into a 2 or 3 liter bottling jar, a china tureen or a glazed earthenware jar (the sort you might use for pickling). If you want to produce larger quantities of the beverage, use a bigger glazed earthenware jar or one or more 5-liter bottling jars. Suppliers of laboratory equipment generally have a wider choice of suitable glass containers in larger sizes. A large glass cooking bowl could be used just as well. This has the additional advantage of providing the large surface area which is needed to promote the process of fermentation. Even a new clean glass aquarium is very suitable and easily obtained. Do not use glass fish tanks with silicone sealer on the inside of the joints. Only use glass bowls that are molded or formed in one piece.

Do not store the tea in painted ceramic containers or vessels made of lead crystal because the tea is acidic and could cause harmful levels of lead to leach into the tea. Don't use any metal or cheap plastic containers. If need be, you could use a high-grade synthetic material of the polyolefin group instead, e.g. polyethylene (PE) or polypropylene. Wine or cider which has a pH value similar to that of kombucha (cider up to around 2.6 pH) is also kept in containers made of this food-grade material. However, you should avoid containers made of polyvinylchloride (PVC) or polystyrene. Styrol can damage your health and can pass from containers made of this material into the liquid undergoing fermentation. Metal is not suitable because the organic acids produced by the kombucha culture can cause a chemical reaction with it.

When making kombucha for the first time, be sure that you get the necessary starter liquid along with the culture, viz. about 0.2 liters (7 ounces) of ready-made kombucha beverage for 2 liters (2 quarts) of tea. For this purpose you can also use kombucha beverage which has fermented for rather longer, viz. some that has gone sour.

If you have received the kombucha culture without the starter liquid from someone, simply add a couple of dessertspoons of vinegar to the tea, boiling the vinegar first if necessary. Use pure white distilled vinegar. Do not use 'live' biological vinegar, as the bacteria in biological vinegar could interfere with the biological components in the kombucha tea culture. The distilled vinegar is added to lower the pH and make the solution acidic to help prevent mold growth in your fermenting k-tea. Henneberg (1926) deems it advisable to use 2 to 4 dessertspoon of boiled vinegar to 1 liter (quart) tea.

The addition of acid at the beginning of the fermentation process, when no acids have yet had time to form, serves to prevent the formation of mold and acts as protection against undesirable microorganism. In the interest of keeping the fermentation process clean, acidification is absolutely necessary.

If you have already made some kombucha beverage, when you make the second and subsequent batches, pour ¼ to ⅛ liters (9-4 oz., equal to 1-½ cup), but in any case at least 10% of ready-made kombucha beverage into the tea (after it has cooled!). This again helps acidification and provides a better start to the process of fermentation.

The Russian scientist L.T. Danielova (1959) recommends acidifying the nutrient solution by means of hydrochloric or acetic acid to a pH value of 5.0-5.5 (Measuring the pH value is discussed in the chapter "When is the beverage ready?") This is apparently a good basis for the fermentation of the antibiotic substances.

You could also add a slice of lemon as they do in Russia. Lakowitz (1928) also recommends putting a slice of lemon into the sweetened tea. The slice of lemon must be thoroughly washed, however, otherwise, destructive microorganisms (mold spores) could appear, which could greatly interfere with growth or even check it. Under such circumstances the skin on the culture grows only very slowly, it at all, and the liquid develops an unpleasant, musty smell instead of its usual typical one (Schmidt, 1979).

No alcohol necessary

Lindner (1917/18) recommends adding a little alcohol to the nutrient solution in some form or other (rum, sherry, port, cognac) right from the outset. Waldeck also (1927) says that the Polish chemist who brewed him the "little miracle drink" in 1915 had asked him for some cognac or rum. The extra shot of alcohol (which is nowadays left out, however) is said to make it possible for the bacteria to begin making acetic acid right away, in case the yeasts which produce alcohol have not yet developed sufficiently in the culture concerned (Steiger and Steinegger, 1957). According to Lindner (1917/1918), when alcohol is added, "it makes the layer of mucilage itself a little more transparent." This can be explained by the fact that the bacteria which produce the gelatinous mass begin their work right away and have a head start on the yeasts which collect in the covering layer.

The Russian research scientist Danielova (1959) conducted some experiments to discover what effects the addition of alcohol has on the nutrient solution. In a special test, it was determined that the acetic bacteria play an active part in the formation of an antibacterial substance in the fermented beverage. To activate these bacteria, 5% ethyl alcohol was slowly added to the nutrient solution as a source of carbon. Danielova mentions at the same time that the nitrogens, which get into the solution through the tea, promote the growth of the yeasts. To clarify the influence of alcohol on the production of antibacterial substances, alcohol was added for purposes of comparison on the 1st, 3rd and 7th day of growth. It was demonstrated that the activity of the nutrient solution was increased by the addition of alcohol at the beginning (1st and 3rd day) of the fermentation process, whereas later additions of alcohol (7th day) produced no increased effectiveness in the nutrient solution.

The kombucha culture
in the nutrient solution

Now put the kombucha culture into the tea solution which is standing in the fermentation container. As you do this, take care (as Mollenda – 1928 – also says) that the layer on the upper surface of the culture is not broken, as otherwise the culture will be considerably weakened.

Why the culture sometimes sinks down and at other times floats on top cannot always be explained. The composition of the water (soft or hard) and that of the culture (e.g. air locked in it) seem to have some part to play in the matter.

When the culture floats on the surface, it initially grows outwards until the surface of the solution is fully covered, and then it grows thicker. The uppermost layer is always the newest. From time to time you can pull off the bottom layer of the membrane so that the culture is constantly rejuvenated. As the culture needs air, the new layer always grows on the upper surface.

If the culture sinks to the bottom, it won't grow there; however, a new culture will begin to form on the surface of the tea. How that happens will be explained in a chapter of its own. A thick glutinous leathery skin begins to form on the surface, at first clear, like water, later on whitish. This skin begins to form by blobs of clear jelly appearing either simultaneously all over the surface of the liquid, or else isolated lumps with a thicker middle and a clear edge are formed first. The whole skin very easily sinks down in one piece, whereupon a new one soon forms on the surface (Henneberg, 1926).

The longer you leave it, the thicker the new culture will grow. The sooner the cover spreads out over the liquid, the sooner you get a sparkling tea, because the cover effectively prevents the escape of carbonic acid (Lindner, 1917/18).

It can also happen that the culture at first sinks down, and then later, as a result of the build-up of carbonic acid, rises to the surface.

The newly formed culture can be used in exactly the same way as the original one. You can put the old culture together with the new one in the same glass. You can thus put as many cultures as you like into one single glass, or else you can start off several larger containers. When the old culture eventually looks rather unsightly after several months (with a brown coating which can't be washed off properly), you can just throw it away, as there are enough new cultures that have grown to take its place.

Many people want to choose for themselves whether the culture sinks or swims. Reasons for this could be that there are too many cultures floating about on the surface, so that no new ones can form; or else you particularly want one specific culture to go on growing on the surface of the tea.

If you want the culture to stay floating on the surface, even though it wants to sink down, then place a couple of corks under it. You could, for instance, use the bread-slicer to cut very thin slices from an ordinary cork, and boil these thoroughly to sterilize them before using them for the first time.

Conversely, if you want the culture to sink down, you need only lay a couple of pebbles on the top, having previously sterilized them in boiling water. Another way is to put a glass marble or a glass on the mother to keep it on the bottom. Then you won't have a problem and the baby will grow fine.

The kombucha culture requires oxygen

The metabolic process of the kombucha culture is dependent on fresh air. Therefore care must be taken that there is always a sufficient supply of oxygen.

For this reason the container should have a wide opening, and the liquid should not lie too far below the lip. A large surface area has a beneficial effect.

Hermann already established in 1928 that large surface areas and shallow liquid depths increase the speed of propagation an acidification. He writes (p. 180): "The speed of propagation and acidification naturally depends on various factors. Large surface areas and a shallow depth of liquid facilitate both processes. For example, if a 5-liter round retort bunged with cotton-wool is used, the same degree of acidification will be reached a few months later than with loosely covered shallow dishes."

The formation of the substances which have an antibacterial effect is also directly dependent on the kombucha culture skin covering the nutrient solution. This is pointed out by the Russian research scientist Sukiasyan (1954). He established that a reduction in the amount of air reaching the surface clearly caused a decrease in activity in the culture fluid, even when the amount of nutrient solution is increased.

The Russian research scientist E. K. Naumova (1949), who writes that the optimum temperature should be 25-30 °C (77-86 °Fahrenheit) as a high concentration of antibiotically effective substances is formed at this level, also mentions that a large surface area has a favorable effect.

In addition, in 1948, Sakaryan and Danielova established that the activity of the kombucha beverage, with respect to the various bacteria, was 2 to 5 times greater in a fermentation container with a large surface area than in a glass retort with a small opening.

This container is optimal:

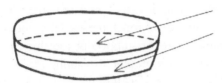

large surface area

shallow depth of liquid
result: speedy propagation
speedy acidification

This container is not so good:

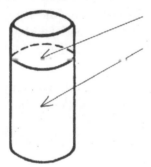

small surface area

deep column of liquid

The fermentation container must be covered

The fermentation container must be covered, as a protection against dust and other particles in the air. Covering it also prevents little vinegar flies, lured by any acid liquid, from laying their eggs on the kombucha culture; white maggots about 5 mm long hatch out of these eggs after a few days. Further details about these pests can be found in the chapter on "Problems."

As a cover you can use a thin layer of muslin or gauze, a piece of net curtain with a very fine mesh, a linen tea-towel or anything similar. A good cover can be made from a tissue. These are generally made of three or four thin layers of paper, and you separate these individual layers and use only one of them as a cover. The weave must not be too open, so that the tiny vinegar flies cannot slip through. For this reason, the cloth must also be securely fastened down either with a rubber band or with a piece of string, so that the little flies cannot possibly crawl through between the cloth and the outside of the container. Airtight stoppers or too thick a cloth should not be used, because they prevent air gaining access. In the hobby magazine "Rund um den Tee" (All About Tea – 1987), covering the container with a household paper towel is also mentioned as a possibility.

Harms (1927) writes that according to the instructions for making given to him by a chemist in Hagen, "the storage jar should be covered with glass, but not completely." Dinslage and Ludorff (1927) covered the container with a watchglass. Mollenda (1928) writes that the container must be covered with a china plate, even though he mentions in the same article that the culture requires air. Precisely because of this need for air, I think covering it with a thin cloth is the most advantageous method.

Influence of light and sun

Light is not required for the process of fermentation, and is even a hindrance. The kombucha culture thrives even in the dark. The container should therefore not stand in bright sunlight, but rather to one side and out of direct light.

We find it confirmed by Mollenda (1928) that apart from warmth, sugar, tea, air and a quiet corner, the kombucha culture requires darkness for healthy growth. And Hermann (1928) established that higher acid content is formed in a darkened container. Here are his results:

Two glass dishes were placed side by side at room temperature. One was covered with transparent paper over the top, the other with black paper stuck down all over.

Contents	Dish exposed to light	Dish without light
10% cane sugar from 12.2 to 7.4 in 50 cc		
volatile acids	38.7 n/2	42.3 n/2
non-volatile acids	16.0	19.0
alcohol	trace	trace

Professor Dittrich (1975, p. 70-71) also writes about the differences in growth between bacteria cultures exposed to light and those left unexposed. After exposure to light and subsequent incubation in an incubator, differences in growth can be seen. Professor Dittrich say: "The growth rate of the surfaces exposed to light is less than that of the darkened ones." From which it can be inferred that "the saying about light, air and sunshine has definitely got something to be said for it. As for our cultures, however, we've come to the conclusion that we should not keep them in brilliant sunlight but rather in a somewhat darker place." Dittrich is talking about bacteria cultures, but his observations could just as well refer to the kombucha culture. It is known to consist partly of bacteria.

And finally, Professor Henneberg (1926, Handbuch der Gärungsbakteriologie – Handbook of Fermentation Bacteriology – Vol. I, p. 6) mentions in his Introduction to Bacteriology that Fungi (which includes the yeasts in the kombucha culture) are "more or less sensitive" to sunlight as well as to ultra-violet light.

The Soviet scientists Sakaryan and Danielova (1948) report that "daylight, the sun's rays and low temperatures" inhibit the vital processes of the kombucha culture, but do not stop them. The metabolism just slows down a bit.

Another Russian article (Roots, 1959) mentions that besides low temperatures, too much sunlight and too many of the sun's rays inhibit the activity of the kombucha culture.

The reason why the kombucha culture dislikes the light could be that sunlight is harmful to certain microorganisms. This is what Schmeil-Seybold (1940, p 379) has to say in the following quotation about the germicidal effect to sunlight, which is certainly desirable in the case of disease germs, but which has an inhibiting effect on the microorganisms in the kombucha culture:

"Natural scientists put clothes, bedding, furniture and other objects, which they had infected with disease germs, out where the sun's rays could reach them, often resulting in the germs being destroyed within just a few hours. In sunlight, particularly in the shortwave range of its spectrum (ultra-violet), we have therefore a disinfectant of a particularly high order." But we should protect our kombucha culture from this 'disinfectant'.

The kombucha culture likes warmth

One of the most important factors in the metabolism and growth of microorganisms is temperature. The individual partners in the kombucha culture symbiosis belong to the so-called mesophyllic type of microorganism, which have a 'normal' temperature. Their optimum development occurs at 20-30 °C (= 68-86 °F), for bacteria, in general, have a higher warmth requirement than yeasts.

Not all the authors who write about kombucha say anything about a particular temperature that helps the culture to thrive. Steiger and Steinegger (1957) state: "Normal room temperature is quite sufficient as a temperature at which culture can become active, although the optimum would lie at a somewhat higher temperature." From my own experience I would agree with this, but I should, nevertheless, like to mention a few other articles.

Henneberg (1926, p. 379) prescribes "**warm room temperature**." Hermann (1928, p. 180) describes the region of 18 to 26 °C (64-79 °F) as the optimum temperature. Reiss (1987, p. 288) names 23-27 °C (73-81 °F) as the optimum growth temperature for the kombucha culture, and found the incubator a good place for it, as this offered the right temperature. Hesseltine (1965, p. 178) used 25 °C (77 °F). E. K. Naumova (1949) pointed out that the optimum temperature is 25-30 °C (77-86 °F) , because at this level a high concentration of antibiotically affective substances can be formed. Bazarewski (1915) worked with a heat of 28 °C (82 °F) and observed rapid growth at this temperature. In a Japanese article by Kozaki (1972) and his colleagues, I read the following statement concerning the bacteria in the kombucha culture: "Opt. tem. 28 °C (82 °F)." Valentin (1928) states that the culture develops best when it is left to stand at a temperature of 30 °C (86 °F). Lakowitz (1928) specifies 30-35 °C (86-95 °F) as the optimum. Bing (1928) writes that the most favorable temperature for the fermentation of the Pombe yeast contained in the kombucha culture, as well as that of the Bacterium xylinum, lies "in the vicinity of bloodheat."

This wide range of temperatures are not only found in the above-mentioned German articles, but also in Russian literature. Barbancik made kombucha beverage for use in his hospital at "the usual temperature" of 20 °C (68 °F). Danielova (1959) on the other hand writes: "The temperature is also quite important for its development. It has been established that most acetic acid bacteria develop best at 28-30 °C (82-86 °F); only with a few does the optimum lie over 30 °C (Bact. aceti Pasterianum, Kützingianum). From the results of our experiments, the best growth of the kombucha culture occurs between 25 and 30 °C. (77-86 °F)"

Nowadays, the ideal temperature that one is likely to find in a normal household without any special facilities for the kombucha culture is generally reckoned to be about 23 °C (73 °F). However, one gathers from the other articles mentioned above that few degrees more or less don't matter. However, the temperature should not sink below 18 °C (64 °F), for then the activity of the bacteria is reduced, and only the yeasts continue to work, as they require less warmth. The consequence of underheating (less 23 °C = 73 °F), as naturopath P. J. Kloucek of Lappersdorf near Regensburg told me, is that you can easily get flatulence from drinking the beverage. On the other hand, at more than 23 °C (73 °F) the bacteria work particularly well; they are responsible, among other things, for the formation of the skin on the culture. By overheating, the skin on the culture becomes gelatinous and slimier. To achieve balanced growth, with bacteria and yeasts functioning equally, you should aim at a temperature of approximately 23 °C (73 °F). Generally one can say that fermentation proceeds quicker at higher temperatures, and the corresponding degree of maturity of the beverage is attained earlier. At lower temperatures the opposite is the case.

Metabolism and growth of the kombucha culture are based on a combination of many chemical processes. It can be derived from the laws of thermodynamics that the speed of chemical reactions increases in proportion to the rise in temperature; in fact a rise in temperature of around 10 °C (= 50 °F) doubles the speed (van't Hoff rule, from Weide and Aurich, 1979).

Sakaryan and Danielova (1948) had noticed that the kombucha culture **develops particularly well during spring and summer**, displaying greater metabolic activity then than in autumn and winter. In spring and summer, the culture forms "a strong mucilaginous mass, and the fluid substance is powerfully effective, whereas growth decreases in autumn and winter." Neither scientist could say why this phenomenon occurs. Temperature differences did not appear to be the sole cause. Although the kombucha culture was kept at the same temperature (25 to 30 °C) in winter, the same results could not be obtained in winter as in spring and summer. When prepared in European homes, the kombucha culture thrives best in summer. The conditions for growth in normal domestic circumstances are in general less favorable in spring because the temperature usually drops at night.

The kombucha culture undoubtedly does best when the optimum temperature remains constant. With a bit of skill, a constant temperature water-bath can be set up with the help of a tub or some other large container and a thermostatically controlled aquarium heater. The fermentation container is placed inside the larger one containing the warm water.

Other requirements of the kombucha culture

The fermentation container should not be moved once the process has been started. Don't carry it around, because otherwise the old skin or the newly forming one can easily sink to the bottom.

You should not smoke in the same room. Apparently, the culture could then dissolve or go moldy.

The kitchen, although often the warmest room in the house, is in my experience not the best place to leave the fermentation container. The frequent variations of a greasy steamy atmosphere have a negative effect.

The fermentation process under way

A succession of complicated biological and chemical metabolic processes takes place in the tea substratum during fermentation, both sequentially and simultaneously. The kombucha culture could be described as a little chemical factory, which, during the time fermentation takes place, produces a small amount of alcohol, carbon dioxide, B vitamins and vitamin C, as well as various organic acids which are important for the human metabolism: acetic acid, gluconic acid, glucuronic acid, lactic acid, oxalic acid and a few others as well.

An inversion of the disaccharides (= compound sugars, such as beet or cane sugar) precedes the processes of forming acids; this means a breakdown into monosaccharides (= simple sugars, such as glucose, fructose, galactose). This division is caused by enzymes and acids. The fermentation process begins with the yeasts converting the sugar into alcohol. This process is represented by a chemical formula thus:

$$C_6 H_{12} O_6 \longrightarrow 2 C_2 H_5 OH + CO_2$$

dextrose   alcohol   carbon dioxide

The carbon dioxide (CO_2) reacts with the moisture in the tea to form carbonic acid:

$$CO_2 + H_2O \longrightarrow H_2CO_3$$

carbon   dioxide   watercarbonic acid

At the same time, the acetic bacteria are building their mucilaginous formation around the kombucha culture. They convert the sugar into cellulose and cause the membrane covering the kombucha culture to gradually grow. At the same time they ferment the alcohol produced by the yeasts into acetic acid and other organic acids. This is an oxidation process, which can be represented thus:

$$C_2 H_5 OH + O_2 \longrightarrow CH_3 CO OH + H_2O$$

alcohol   oxygen   acetic acid   water

The acidification of the sweetened tea is therefore caused by the metabolic activity of the microorganisms in the kombucha culture. The speed of acidification depends on how favorable the vital conditions are which are provided for the organisms. The deciding factors are: the composition of the symbiotic culture (according to Dinslage and Ludorff, 1927, this is not always constant; conditions are sometimes more favorable for this type of yeast, sometimes for that, sometimes for the acetic bacteria); size and shape of the fermentation container, and in particular, the amount of surface expansion this allows; the extent to which oxygen can gain access; the composition of the air (pollution?); the quality of the water; what the tea is like; how much sugar there is, and what kind; and above all, the temperature. Due to the varying factors, the acidification process is not always the same.

During the course of the fermentation process, the beverage develops a pleasantly sharp aromatic odor. The color becomes lighter on account of the increasing acidity. Through the development of the yeasts the beverage can become a little cloudy. Little frothy bubbles of gas develop here and there. This is to do with the carbon changing into carbonic acid as a result of the moisture in the tea. It also frequently happens that a bubble of carbonic gas gets caught under the skin on the surface of the liquid and lifts it up at that particular spot so that the rest of the skin hangs down like a curtain all the way round and makes the kombucha culture look almost like a jellyfish.

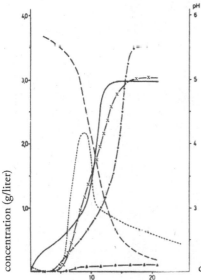

How the contents develop during the course of the fermentation process is very clearly seen in the results of Dr. Jürgen Reiss's investigations.

(From Deutsche Lebens-mittelrundschau – German Food Review), 83rd year, No. 9, 1987, with kind permission of the publisher and author.)

Substances contained in kombucha made from black tea:

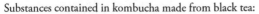

————— lactic acid   –x–x– gluconic acid
– ▲ – ▲ – acetic acid   –·–·– ethanol
·············· glucose   – – – pH value

The Frankish Continuous Fermentation

Instead of what is simply known as continuous fermentation, I would recommend the "Frankish Continuous Fermentation." It is convenient and time-saving. The difference is that rather than "harvesting" or filling up with new tea on a daily basis, you do it every 10 to 15 days. By doing so, you save yourself having to make tea daily. In contrast to continuous fermentation, you harvest a ready fermented beverage and not a mix of ready beverage and sugared tea.

Here is the method: Use a fermenting container with an outlet tap e.g. a drinks barrel. Once a fermentation process is complete, transfer it to glass bottles via the outlet tap. At least 10% should stay in the fermenting container with the mushroom and sediment as starting liquid for the next batch. Fill it up with fresh tea. It suffices if you take the mushroom out every few months and clean the inside of the barrel. Should the beverage be too tart for you, remove the sediment more often.

Part 5
Harvesting and drinking

When is the kombucha beverage ready?

The acidification process, as already mentioned, is dependent on several factors and does not always proceed in the same way. Furthermore, people seem to have very different ideas as to when the beverage is ready. Hans Irion in his "Lehrgang für Drogistenfachschulen" (Training Course for Pharmaceutical Technical Colleges – 1944) recommends a fermentation period of 5 to 6 days. Other authors decree from 8 to 10 days, and yet others from 10 to 12 or 10 to 14 days for the period of fermentation. Ingeborg Oetinger (1988), who considers the acid/alkali problem to be crucial, thinks one should only let the beverage get slightly sour. Dr. Reiss (1987) mentions that tea kvass made from black tea possessed a particularly pleasant taste after an incubation period of 6 days. After 10 days, the vinegar taste predominated.

Dinslage and Ludorff (1927) write: "Whereas, after three days the taste of the tea kvass was pleasantly like fruit juice, after 14 days an unpleasantly strong, sour, and only slightly aromatic taste was evident. Further, after 3 days, the following could be detected: 0.33 % alcohol, 0.06 % volatile acid (acetic acid), 0.11 % non-volatile acid (lactic acid), and 2.02 % acid in all, as against the following after 14 days: 0.73 alcohol, 0.25 % volatile acid, 0.35 % non-volatile acid, and 8.10 % acid all told. The drinkability of the tea kvass seemed from these results to be at its best after about three days to at most six days of activity by the kombucha culture. When made in this way, the drink is mildly tangy, has a pleasant smell, an in the first few days of the fermentation process, allows both the smell and the taste of the tea to come through quite distinctly, whereas after a longer period of fermentation the acid character of the beverage comes to the fore too much and prohibits the consumption of any great quantities."

Mollenda (1928) writes thus in an article: "In Winter, the teas must be poured off after 5-6 days, in Summer after 3-4 days. Before doing so, the kombucha culture must first be lifted out and laid on a clean china plate; then the beverage can be filled into bottles, corked, and kept in a cool place for a further 3-6 days before drinking."

Lindner (197/18) even writes about preparing the kombucha beverage by means of a two-day fermentation: "Liquid and culture should be taken out every 2 days, and the latter washed clean with lukewarm water before being put back again into a fresh infusion of tea sweetened with sugar (1 soupspoon of sugar to ½ a liter of tea), the container having in the meantime been cleaned out. Two-day tea-kvass comes out as a fairly clear, very slightly sour beverage with an aroma reminiscent of a Moselle wine and with a slight sparkle. Guests are always very happy to drink it, on account of this quality."

A German lady living in Russia even told me that her mother used to brew tea daily and place the kombucha culture in it for just the one day. The very next day the tea would be drunk as a household beverage by the whole family.

Personally, I used to leave the tea to ferment mostly for 12 to 14 days, so that the sugar would be thoroughly converted. The beverage is then similar in taste to a well-fermented dry wine without much residual sweetness, and it doesn't taste too wonderful, either, but is easier to digest. However, kombucha that has been fermented for 14 days is not to everyone's taste. My wife protested at the acidity which in her opinion was too strong. Since then, I pour the beverage off after about 8 to 10 days. If the taste is more important to you, or you have to have some consideration for your family's taste buds (after all, they have to drink the beverage, too), then I recommend that you begin with a fermentation period of about 8 days. You may gradually increase the fermentation period to 14 days if your family accepts the sourer taste.

There is a point in favor of a fermentation period of 8 days which I've found lacking in the German articles about kombucha, but, which has been given the greatest attention in Russian research – the kombucha infusion has antibiotic qualities. The research work done by Sakaryan and Danielova (Professor and Lecturer respectively at the Institute for Zoological and Veterinary Science, Yerevan) has shown that the activity which is necessary for the destruction of bacteria occurs on the 7th and 8th day. The exact time depends of course on the amount of sugar and the temperature, which are not mentioned in the article I have to hand (Roots, 1959).

The Scientific Director of the hospital at the Water Transport Works in Omsk, Professor G. Barbancík (1958) and his colleagues has been doing research since 1949 on the treatment of several diseases by means of the kombucha beverage. They used 50 g of sugar per liter, and established that the infusion reached its highest state of activity after the 7th to the 8th day, at a normal temperature of 20 °C. They therefore gave their patients kombucha which had been fermented for 8 days (with success, as reported below). So that a fresh supply of the beverage would be available every day, they cultivated the tea in 7 or 8 containers, filling one container anew every day.

The individual period of fermentation will be a compromise between how highly each person rates the factors of residual sugar, degree of acidity, personal taste, and the antibiotic elements mentioned in the Russian articles.

I mention the varying views about the period of fermentation in such detail so you can see that there really is a great deal of scope. It would be insincere to set out some sort of a rule that would be applicable to all. It depends on personal taste and on how each individual person's body reacts. In the end, **each person can regulate the degree of acidity** as they find best, depending on their own circumstances and requirements. This isn't the same for everybody.

When the beverage is ready, it has (as Mollenda writes, 1928) "a yellow amber color and a sweet-sour wine-must flavor, in which the sharp taste should predominate." This, however, depends principally on what kind of teas has been used. With rose-hip tea, the beverage naturally doesn't have a yellow amber color but a reddish one. Even the culture in this case acquires a reddish hue.

The degree of acidity of the kombucha beverage is expressed in terms of pH value. A pH value of 7 is called neutral. With a value under 7 there is an acid reaction, with a value over 7 a basic or alkaline reaction. The pH value of the fermented kombucha beverage lies between 2.5 and 4, depending on the degree of fermentation. In cases where the culture is dying off, the liquid has a neutral or alkaline reaction and smells foul.

To measure the pH value, you use things called indicators which are either paper strips, measuring strips or fluid indicators. The indicators take on a particular coloring according to the pH value, which you then compare with a color chart. The fluid indicators react the quickest. The strip indicators are simpler to handle, but it can sometimes take a long time till they stop changing color. There are also electronic pH meters, but they are very expensive.

The jump between one pH value and another – as for example between pH value 4 and 3 – means that the solution is 10 times more acid. The greater the range measured by the indicators, the larger the levels. An indicator, with a scale from 1 to 14 pH, can at the most determine pH differences of 1 to 2 units. Such indicators naturally give very inaccurate results.

If we want to measure the degree of acidity of the kombucha beverage (the taste test is too inaccurate), a measurement range of 2.5 to 5 pH is enough as a rule. For this range, there are a number of indicators graded in values of 0.2 to 0.5 pH unit degrees which are available from chemists and shops selling laboratory requisites. The following are very suitable for measuring the pH value of kombucha:

- pH universal indicator in roll form (4.8m),
  range pH 1.0 – 10.0 by 1 pH unit degrees
- pH universal indicator (100 strips),
  range pH 1.0 – 14.0 by 1 pH unit degrees

- Acilite indicator (100 strips),
  range pH 0 – 6.0 by 0.5 degrees
- pH special indicator (100 strips),
  range pH 2.5 – 4.5 by 0.2 – 0.3 degrees

The beverage won't always be the same. There are fluctuations in flavor, and there are variations in appearance. When the beverage is ready it sometimes tingles slightly on the tongue, and little bubbles of carbonic acid sparkle upwards. Or the little bubbles of carbonic acid might be almost entirely absent or might only develop once the beverage is bottled. I found these often inexplicable fluctuations confirmed in an article by List and Hufschmidt (1959), who write: "In tests that we carried out with the kombucha culture, we observed that a strong formation of CO_2 took place in many of the vessels containing the culture, whereas in others which were prepared with the same kombucha culture, relatively little CO_2 was developed, although we had kept all the cultures under the same conditions."

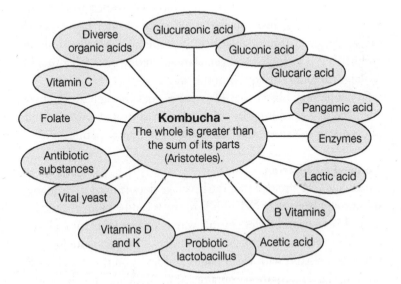

So don't worry if the beverage doesn't always turn out the same for you either. With a living organism such variations are normal.

We can all have our own preferences when it comes to taste so it is laudable to try and give an account of your individual taste. If the beverage becomes too acidic during the usual fermentation period (8 to 12 days), try the following: Cover the container with a plate for a while (in addition to the fabric cover). As a result, the fungus gets less air. Those microorganisms that produce the milder lactic acid work more, so the drink is less acidic.

Drawing off and bottling the beverage

For a while, I used coffee filter papers to filter the beverage when it was ready. The beverage will be almost clear if you use that method. Any residual bits and pieces will be caught by the filter paper. This gets clogged up very quickly and has to be renewed frequently when straining off larger amounts. So for some time I experimented with folded filters. For this, you fold a big piece of filter paper (which can be obtained from a chemist's) in a special concertina fashion, and when it is unfolded you get a larger filtering area. Chemists filter larger amounts of liquids in this way.

Someone may object that filter paper goes through an intensive chemical process during its production. It is treated with all kinds of chemicals to achieve stability at the same time as permeability.

No need for filtering
Since then, I've decided that the beverage doesn't need to be filtered so thoroughly anyway. When it is ready, it can be poured quite un-filtered into clean bottles. In this way it retains its natural cloudiness. You take the kombucha culture out of the fermentation container beforehand with clean hands and lay it on a clean plate. By holding the fermentation container at an angle or with the help of a ladle you pour the liquid through a sieve (which catches the worst

of the impurities) and through a funnel into the bottles. You can also leave the kombucha culture in the fermentation container and pour off the liquid by tilting the container carefully at an angle, leaving just a little to leaven the new infusion. Or you can insert a thin tube into the container, suck the liquid up through the tube, and so siphon off the beverage.

Sediment is good for the intestines

Don't be worried if a piece of the yeast sediment gets into the bottled beverage. It is considered that certain yeast cells have a beneficial effect on the gastro-intestinal tract, normalize the intestinal bacteria, and through immune stimulation of the intestine contribute to the unspecific increase in resistance to disease. The yeast Saccharomyces cerevisiae Hansen CBS 5926 for example has recently been used as a drug (Perenterol) because of its immunological effect. According to an article in the Ärzte-Zeitung (Medical Times) of 10.04.89 the yeast cells are suitable both as prophylaxis as well as therapy for intestinal diseases. According to Professor K. D. Tympner of Munich, "the immunogenic potency of yeast cells" has definitely been verified in recent times. According to a statement by Professor Jürgen Hotz of Celle, the yeast cells release a whole series of substances throughout the intestinal tract, which may encourage the growth of apathogenic bacteria and may have an antagonistic (hostile) effect against facultative pathogenic (disease-causing) bacteria. Even though it is still not known exactly how the yeast therapy mechanism works, it may be assumed that the yeast cells in the kombucha beverage have similar mechanisms which are equally effective, as with the yeast Saccharomyces cerevisiae Hansen CBS 5926 mentioned in the article in the Ärzte-Zeitung. This yeast is being used in experiments to see if even diseases with chronic inflammation of the intestine (Crohn's disease) can be influenced through alteration of the bacteria in the intestinal tract. (Reference: Ärzte-Zeitung 8, 64, p. 16, 10.04.89)

New streaky jelly-like bits may form in the filled bottles. Mollenda (1928) speaks of "light and dark brown algae". In my opinion, they are offshoots which have formed from little pieces of the kombucha culture which slipped through when the beverage was being bottled. To prevent these pieces from getting into the beverage when it is poured out for drinking, it should again be filtered through a sieve as it goes into the glass. Mollenda recommends "straining the beverage through a clean linen cloth before drinking". I consider a sieve to be better because the larger pieces are held back but the yeasts pass through.

From time to time (every four weeks) the sediment at the bottom of the container, which makes the beverage cloudy and mostly consists of pure yeast culture, must be removed by rinsing out the container with water. Henneberg (1926) recommends this, and adds: "If you like a greater amount of carbonic acid and not such a sharp tang, you must stimulate the growth of the yeasts and inhibit the formation of acids by the vinegar culture. This occurs by frequently pouring off the tea and infrequently removing the sediment, because the yeasts for the most part accumulate in this." The yeasts in the sediment are responsible for a speedy start to the new fermentation process.

Wash the mushroom before using it again

After bottling the beverage, you can begin to prepare the new brew. Before doing so, you should wash the kombucha culture under running lukewarm or cold water. Mollenda recommends giving the culture a good soak before starting it off anew. He describes it in this way: "In Winter, the culture should not be soaked in a water-bath at all; in summer it should be soaked once every 4–6 weeks in lukewarm water (...) for five minutes, and after letting it drip dry, it should be placed in a freshly made infusion of tea that has been allowed to cool down to lukewarm."

According to Henneberg, "when the tea kvass is ready, and tastes something like a cider or a dry white wine, if it is not going to be used right away, it should be kept as cool as possible in bottles filled right to the top to prevent further acidification and culture growth." On the basis of personal experience, I prefer not to fill the bottles right to the top, as the beverage can continue to work even in bottles filled right to the top, and through the build-up of carbonic acid, excess pressure develops which can cause the bottles to burst. For this reason, I prefer to use bottles which can be corked, so that if excess pressure builds up, the cork can be pulled out in an emergency.

As Henneberg also mentions, it can quite easily happen that a new little kombucha culture forms within the bottle on the surface of the beverage, if the bottle has been left standing for some time. That is no drawback however, and it proves the adaptability of the culture and how undemanding it is, that although it actually requires oxygen, it can form a baby culture purely from the offshoots contained in the already fermented beverage.

Keep cool for long storage

Once the bottles are filled, they should be stored in a cool place, preferably in the fridge or in a cool cellar, so as to keep the secondary fermentation within bounds. When stored in this way, the beverage can be kept for a long time. The acid prevents it from going bad. Sakaryan and Danielova (1948) established that the effectiveness of the kombucha beverage gradually decreases during storage over a longer period of time, nevertheless, even after 5 months, does not completely disappear and is even then quite big. The longer the beverage remains in the bottle, the better it tastes, because it keeps on working. The beverage should be allowed to stand for three to six days after bottling, and before beginning to drink it. Carbonic acid builds up through secondary fermentation, and it can only escape when the bottle is opened. The carbonic acid gives an effervescent, refreshing character to the beverage. Just let a glass of kombucha slide over your tongue, and allow the rising bubbles of carbonic acid to tickle your palate, just as wine-drinkers do – it's a truly refreshing thirst-quencher, and a healthy one at that.

The bottle in current use does not need to be kept in the fridge, of course; the beverage can be kept at room temperature, which is better for the stomach. The beverage may also be diluted with warm water. However, if it is heated to more than 40 °C (for instance, if you want to make mulled wine with kombucha), the yeast cells which have slipped through into the beverage will be destroyed. Other substances, such as glucuronic acid or the antibiotic substances, will not be affected even by heating to 100 °C.

Stimulating effects are increased

A chemist gave me a good tip and told me to add about 1 gram (about the tip of a teaspoon) of ascorbic acid (Acidum ascorbicum) when bottling the beverage. Ascorbic acid is vitamin C in pure crystalline form. It is an anti-oxidant, and can be obtained at every chemist's. The quality of the beverage is thereby enhanced, and it keeps for longer.

There was an interesting suggestion made in "Hobbythek: Rund um den Tee" (Hobbytique: All About Tea), 1987, though it has the disadvantage of a higher sugar content. In the Hobbythek Tips, which among other things deal with making kombucha, it states: "It's also possible to use bottles with metal caps (such as beer bottles or mineral water bottles) and leave it to ferment again for a few more days. You could even add ½ to 1 teaspoon of sugar per 0.7 liter bottle before putting the caps on, so that the yeasts in the tea kvass which cause the slight cloudiness can work a bit more for 3 to 4 days. The alcohol content of the beverage will thereby be fractionally increased, and further amounts of carbon dioxide will be released, which is what gives the beverage its refreshing effect."

Blend in fruits

To add a bit of variety to the taste, I'll pass on a couple of tips for you to try out. Valentin (1928) writes in the Apotheker-Zeitung (Pharmaceutical Times) that he obtained a particularly pleasant smelling liquid when he "added small amounts of preserved fruit (cranberry, apple, raspberry, etc.). In the first place, the culture found ample nourishment from the nitrogenous substances contained in the fruit, and then the aromatic substances in the fruit imparted their flavor to the solution."

Note that Valentin used preserved fruit. It is not advisable to let fresh, uncooked fruit ferment with the liquid. You then run the risk of introducing unwanted bacteria and wild yeasts into the culture.

Fresh, uncooked fruit can in fact be used, but it should only be added once the beverage is ready for bottling, that is, when the fermentation process has finished. I add a few raspberries now and then to the beverage when it is ready for bottling, or a few cherries, blackberries, etc. – whatever happens to be available in the garden at the time. The beverage takes on a hint of the fruit flavor and acquires a different coloring for a change. Or try pushing a couple of fresh elderflower heads down the neck of the bottle and into the beverage. That way, the tea acquires an especially characteristic delicate dry taste which always reminds me of the "elderflower champagne" my grandmother used to make when the elderflower was in bloom.

A teacher told me that after she has bottled the beverage, she drops a dessertspoon of raisins into the bottle. The beverage then ferments again, and acquires a particularly delicious taste through the leaching of the raisins. This idea is also to be found in many old Russian recipes for making kvass, in which time and again one is advised to drop one to three raisins into the bottle before filling it with the fermented kvass.

Through such variations and experiments, you can add variety to the taste and thus avoid boredom gradually setting in and dulling the pleasure of drinking the beverage. However, do note that you must only add such things to the finished, fermented beverage, so that no unwanted bacteria get in.

There are many paths
to the top of the mountain,
but the view is always the same.

(Chinese saying)

How much kombucha should one drink, and when?

The beverage was originally chiefly enjoyed as a refreshing drink, on account of its aromatic taste similar to that of cider or fruit wine. In many areas it was called "tea kvass." It got this name from a product that is widely known and loved in Russia, called "kvass." The word "kvass" comes from the Russian and virtually means "acid." Professor Lindner (1917/18) describes the fermented beverage kvass as a slightly sour, weak beer, which in Russia is made from rye flour and malt or from bran and flour or from black bread and apples, which are left to ferment in water, and to which various other ingredients are added. The acid contained in kvass is primarily lactic acid which, as is well known, has a beneficial effect on the digestive system. In Russian military hospitals, writes Prof. Lindner, nearly every patient receives a liter (= 1.057 quarts) of kvass daily.

Even though the acids in kombucha are of a different sort, and even though the beverage does not contain the same constituent elements as the Russian kvass, it is natural and understandable that in the absence of another term, the name "kvass" was conferred on the kombucha beverage as well.

A glass several times a day
Apart from being a refreshing drink, tea kvass, that is to say kombucha, has been highly prized for centuries as a household remedy for all sorts of illnesses. The many publications on this subject mention this time and again.

In extensive world literature, there are few directions to be found as to how much kombucha you should drink, and when. One of the few authors to give more precise advice about drinking kombucha is Dr. Mollenda. In 1928, he wrote: " ½ to ¾ liter (18 to 26 ounces) a day is the recommended dosage, to be taken in the following manner: the beverage should be strained and drunk cool two or three times a day, after the midday meal and after the evening meal, possibly also after breakfast, ¼ liter (9 ounces) each time."

In 1944, Hans Irion, who was at that time the director of the state-recognized Pharmaceutical Academy in Brunswick, Germany, gave the following directions: "One should drink 1 or 2 wine glasses full a day, on an empty stomach in the morning, and after the midday and evening meal. It tastes marvelous, slightly sharp, almost like a light dry white wine." This recommendation of Iron's was then taken over almost word for word by Dr. Sklenar. According to Fasching (1988), as part of his additional therapy, Dr. Sklenar prescribed, 3 x ¼ liter (= 3 x 9 ounces) of kombucha (+ Mutaflor capsules) a day, and according to other sources, ½ liter (18 ounces) a day, for the treatment of precancer (the preliminary stage of cancer). The program of treatment for established cancer included a liter of kombucha a day (plus kombucha drops, Mutaflor capsules, Gelum oral rd (+) drops and Colibiogen ampoules).

Kraft (1959) recommends drinking a glass of the beverage every morning on an empty stomach. The amount drawn off should immediately be replaced with fresh sugared tea. I also found this recommendation (to remove the required amount each day and replace it at once with the same amount of fresh tea) in some other publications as well, e.g. in the directions for use issued by the Chemical and Bacteriological Laboratory of the Yeast Institute, Kitzingen, mentioned by Arauner (1929). Bing (1928) also recommends drinking some of the fermenting liquid several times a day, and each day making up the amount of tea drawn off. I don't like the idea of this method, due to the great quantities of unfermented sugar present in the solution as a result of this.

Local consumers in Russia, Japan, India, etc. apparently only drink ⅓ liter (12 ounces) a day. I'm inclined to recommend this amount because the positive effects noted by the people of these nations are based on this dosage. If you want to adhere to this recommendation, drink 0.1 liter (about 4 ounces) 3 times a day – that is, one glass in the morning on an empty stomach, about 10-15 minutes before breakfast, one glass before or after the midday meal, and the last glass in the evening some time before going to bed.

You can regard this recommendation as a rule of thumb to begin with. It's a guideline, but there's no need to stick to it. You should find out for yourself what the best dosage for your own needs is. Each person is unique, with their own constitution and sensibilities and individual biological predisposition. I know of some people who only drink 3 liqueur glasses a day. There are others who feel great drinking larger quantities, between meals as well.

Why should the first glass be taken in the morning on an empty stomach, but the other glasses after meals? I presume that by recommending this dosage, Irion and Dr. Sklenar wanted to cover as broad a range of effectiveness as possible, using the great variety of substances contained in kombucha. It is known in pharmacology that absorption of certain active substances into the bloodstream or lymph stream is reduced if taken before meals, e.g. certain fungicides. On the other hand, other active substances should be taken on an empty stomach, e.g. antibiotics. Now kombucha contains a great number of substances.

The small amounts of **antibiotic substances** contained in kombucha are rendered especially effective when the beverage is taken in the morning on an empty stomach, whereas, for example the organic acids stimulate a better functioning of the digestive processes when the beverage is taken after the more ample midday and evening meals. But as I've already said, I don't see any need to be particularly dogmatic about the above-mentioned recommendations. Our body is a good barometer if we understand how to recognize its reactions and interpret them correctly. For instance, my wife says it would give her "gooseflesh inside" if she had to drink a glass of kombucha before breakfast. So she drinks her first glass during the course of the morning on a partly empty stomach. However, the first thing I do after I get up in the morning is to drink a glass of kombucha, and despite our different ways of taking it, we both feel well.

Mollenda (1928) writes: "The beneficial effects of kombucha, even in serious and long-term cases, regularly become apparent after 4 to

6 weeks of continuous consumption." I have heard of several people who already noticed positive effects on their general well-being after a much shorter time, e.g. after two days. On the other hand, other kombucha users report that the sometimes astonishing effect only begins to show after taking it continuously over a period of one or two years. Generally speaking, it's necessary to take it over an extended period of time.

The interval method

A doctor suggested another theory to me, that the right thing to do might be to take kombucha for e.g. two months and then stop for an interval of one month, to prevent addiction to the stimulation setting in. Everything needs a stimulus, but continual stimulation becomes tiring. This interval theory, however, is for the time being just a working hypothesis, and I mention it purely for the sake of completeness.

The following observation is the basis for the theory mentioned above: it was noted even in olden times that repeatedly taking frequent doses of various substances lessened their effectiveness. The strength of the effect decreases and at the same time the period of effectiveness becomes shorter. To achieve the original effectiveness again, the dose has to be increased or the substance taken more frequently. You could call this phenomenon a sort of de-sensitizing, a rendering insensitive. This addictive habit effect, however, does not work in the same way for all substances. There are substances whose effectiveness diminishes when taken over a long period of time, but there are others where the effectiveness remains constant, independent of the dosage. To my knowledge, there has not been sufficient research done on this aspect of kombucha. I personally can't go along with the interval theory because I don't want to miss out on my daily drink of kombucha. I know of people who have been drinking kombucha for years and who enjoy the best of good health.

Can diabetics drink kombucha?

Dr. Mollenda (1928) writes as follows in answer to this question: "Those persons afflicted with diabetes can, according to the expert opinion of doctors, drink well-fermented kombucha as well as sour milk or sour cream, because the sugar, which for the most part is contained in the tea, is broken down into its component parts and converted by the process of fermentation."

By chance, I heard the suggestion that diabetics could drink kombucha, but that they should dilute it with herbal tea or mineral water. Then the amount of sugar (residual sugar) absorbed into the system would be negligible, so long as the permitted total amount of sugar within the limits of the dietary prescription is not exceeded. Because fully fermented kombucha tea is too sour for most people, you should aim to get a residual sugar proportion of about 25 to 30 grams per liter, provided that 100 grams of sugar were used as starting sugar.

The residual sugar contained in the tea, however, consists for the most part only of fructose, which is allowed in some measure even to diabetics. The reason for this is that white sugar (saccharose, a disaccharide) splits at the beginning of the fermentation process, by the action of the enzymes in the yeast and the acetobacters, into the simple sugars glucose and fructose. The glucose ferments quicker and more easily.

The fructose remains as residual sugar, which is converted slower and with greater difficulty. This can also be concluded from the experiments by Reiss (1987), who established that the glucose concentration rose rapidly from the 5th to the 9th day (because of the splitting), but then on account of the metabolic processes which break down the glucose, quickly decreased. On the 17th day the reserves of glucose were nearly exhausted.

As a possible way of achieving as small an amount of residual sugar as possible, it is also under discussion whether or not as little sugar as possible should be used when starting off the beverage, and that the beverage should then be left to ferment thoroughly (three to four weeks). To soften the rough taste, the really quite sour end product can be diluted before drinking, or if necessary, sweetened with a synthetic sweetener. In the article which follows later, Dr. Abele considers just 40 grams of sugar per liter to be sufficient. In my opinion, a minimum of 70 g/liter should be used. One has to realize that the less sugar available to the kombucha culture as nutriment and starting material, the less the desired substances can be formed which have a positive effect on your health.

I believe the microorganisms in the kombucha culture will be undernourished if they receive too little sugar, and the culture will degenerate. I don't consider it so important to use a small amount of starting sugar when aiming for a low residual sugar content, but that it's vital to let the sugar be converted into the various metabolic products through a sufficiently long period of fermentation.

Drink kombucha and keep moving

Dr. Johann Abele, Medical Director of the Sanatorium for Natural Methods of Healing, Schloss Lindach, Schwäbisch Gmünd, offers advice which can be of help to diabetics who are trying to make up their minds. From the holistic approach of a doctor advocating natural methods of healing, he gives the following answer to a reader's question, whether as a latent diabetic, she could drink the "Kombucha culture beverage" (Answers to reader's questions in "Der Naturarzt" (The Naturopath), 128th year, No. 12/88, p. 31): "Latent diabetes is a gerontic diabetes and a dietetic problem. If you adhere strictly dietetically to the guidelines laid down by the old masters such as Kollath or Bircher-Benner, kombucha tea should make no difference. In addition to this, you should get plenty of movement, indeed, more than "other people". Then if you have fulfilled the above-mentioned requirements, you can even drink kombucha tea. Like the full diabetic, the latent diabetic is an acid patient. The acid balance of the body has to be equalized. Then you will be able to even tolerate kombucha perfectly well. Usually people drink too much of it, however. One glassful a day is perfectly adequate. kombucha can be prepared with absolutely less sugar than you write. 80 g sugar to about two liters of tea is sufficient. The kombucha culture works on the sugar so that basically no residual sugar remains. It contains several acids, however, including lactose among others, which in the case of a diseased intestine does not improve the acidity level of the intestinal tract for one thing, but makes it worse. The type of sugar you use makes little difference. You can use honey, unrefined whole cane sugar, fructose, dextrose or normal granulated sugar." (Der Naturarzt, Heft 12/88, p. 31).

In the Allos honey brochure (Allos GmbH, Imkerhof, D-49457 Drebber), I found the following tip, which, assuming that this information is tenable, suggests that diabetics should use honey when they make kombucha: "Honey differs from pure sugar in one further essential point, and that is with regard to the metabolic disease diabetes mellitus. This disease causes the blood sugar level to be raised on account of a relative or absolute lack of insulin. Blood sugar diagrams have shown that the blood sugar level can be lowered to a normal state by the intravenous administration of honey. Clinical tests have shown that the more serious the diabetes, the more strongly marked the regulating effect of the honey on the blood sugar level is. The effect is primarily ascribed to the substance choline contained in the honey (Baumgarten and Koch, Theoretische Medizin (Theoretical Medicine), Ärztliche Forschung (Medical Research I/528). Hence for diabetic therapy, there arise aspects which must emphatically be taken into consideration in the treatment of diabetes."

Individual levels of tolerance

I am mentioning this information for the sake of completeness, to show what theories are being discussed. I would not like to judge whether this recommendation to use honey is scientifically tenable. Normally, honey is forbidden for diabetics (Mehnert and Förster, 1970). If I were a diabetic, I would be cautious. By keeping a check on their blood sugar, diabetics should ascertain whether any changes occur through drinking kombucha. It is a known fact that each diabetic has their own individual tolerance limit; that means that with the help of the remaining functions of their insulin glands, they can convert a limited amount of carbohydrate without the blood sugar rising dangerously (Schneidrzik, 1985).

As diabetics can use certain sugars or sugar alcohol to prepare their food, the use of e.g. fructose instead of white saccharose sugar also requires consideration, as this produces a metabolism that is largely independent of insulin (Mehnert and Förster, 1970, p. 204), and is therefore recommended as a diabetic sugar. According to Mehnert and Förster, fructose is, in general, well tolerated even by diabetics if it is spread over the day in small portions, and in appropriate cases it can be administered in doses of up to 60 g a day.

Fructose is therefore supposedly tolerated by diabetics because the greater part of it is transported directly to the liver without causing the blood sugar level to rise. Fructose does not itself stimulate the release of insulin, though insulin is required for its resorption.

Resolute opponents of sugar, such as Dr. Bruker, consider any kind of manufactured sugar unsuitable for diabetics. By "manufactured sugar", we understand any kind of sugar which is produced in a factory. Isolated fructose counts as one of these. Dr. Bruker (1989, p. 92) writes: "All types of manufactured sugar are unsuitable for diabetics. Not even fructose" and (p. 94) "isolated fructose should be strictly avoided by diabetics."

Different forms of sugar – different fermentation results
Several scientists have conducted experiments in which they substituted other types of sugar for cane sugar (saccharose), and tested how these react during the fermentation process of kombucha. I have compared the results obtained by Henneberg (1926), Hermann (1928) and Wiechowski (1928), in so far as the authors give details about the various types of sugar:

– Cane sugar
Henneberg: "is mostly acidified."
Hermann: "is converted into gluconic acid and acetic acid."
Wiechowski: "acetic acid and gluconic acid are produced in nearly equal amounts."

– Chemically pure glucose
Hermann: "is for the most part converted into gluconic acid."
Wiechowski: "produces almost exclusively gluconic acid."

– Mannitol (besides glucose and fructose, contained in manna from 70 to 90%, in poor qualities often only 30%, according to Hager, 1970)
Henneberg: "is very little acidified."
Hermann: "is not altered."

–Fructose (levulose)
Henneberg: "is very slightly acidified."
Hermann: "levulose produces almost exclusively acetic acid. The proportion of volatile acids is infinitesimally small. Gluconic acid could not be detected in any instance. The skins that are formed are very thick and yellowish white, and bear bud-like outgrowths."
Wiechowski: "almost exclusively acetic acid is produced."

– Lactose and maltose
All three authors are unanimous that these types of sugar are not, or almost not acidified. Despite ample growth of the culture or favorable growth of the bacteria, no corresponding acids are produced.

Danielova (1954), who, after a long series of experiments, came to the conclusion that the metabolic products of the kombucha culture have an antibacterial effect, also tested several types of sugar. The Russian author established that "the accumulation of antibacterial substances is greater on substrata with glucose and saccharose" and less marked on substrate with levulose, although the latter is fermented well by the yeasts.

As we can see from all of these results, the fructose which is suitable for diabetics is used by the yeast as well as by the bacterial components of the kombucha culture, but it produces almost exclusively acetic acid and not the desired gluconic acid nor the antibacterial substances.

Anyone who wants to experiment with fructose in spite of these not very encouraging reports should bear in mind that fructose takes longer to ferment than glucose (Belitz and Grosch, 1985, p. 696). The period of fermentation must therefore be extended in comparison with the use of cane sugar.

Kombucha drops

Today, diabetics are advised to take mainly the so-called "kombucha drops" instead of the kombucha beverage. Other terms are also used instead of the term "kombucha drops", but I should like to use this expression for the sake of simplicity. Kombucha drops are also recommended for non-diabetics, as they are said to have a stronger effect.

The first reference to the production of kombucha in a concentrated form comes from Wiechowski (1928) and Hermann (1929). Hermann regarded it as essential to have a preparation made up according to the principles of the cultivation of pure cultures, and of unvarying composition, so as to be able to draw comparisons. The Norgine Pharmaceutical Works in Prague-Aussig declared themselves willing to produce an experimental preparation made up to Hermann's prescription. This preparation was then distributed to chemists' shops under the name "Kombuchal". "Kombuchal" (German Reichspatent 538 028) was made from a culture liquid that was fermented to a specific degree of acidity and reduced to a specific concentration by means of vacuum distillation. It contained all the substances produced by the kombucha culture except for acetic acid and alcohol, which no doubt evaporated as easily liquefied component elements together with the aqueous part.

Hermann and a series of doctors at the "Clinic for Internal Medicine" in Prague, all worked with this preparation. Hermann writes that the doctors at the clinic commented on the extraordinarily favorable effects, but adds: "Although all those who tested it, be they clinicians or general practitioners, can testify to rally favorable effects on symptoms of senility and on arteriosclerosis and the symptoms connected with it, they nevertheless hesitate to publish, just because folk remedy is encumbered with a certain prejudice."

The kombucha drops available commercially today are described by the manufacturers either as elixir or as pressed extract. The latter term gives a clue as to the manufacturing process. Apart from that, the manufacturers pursue an information policy of great reticence about the way their preparations are made.

The idea of pressing the kombucha culture seems to stem from Dr. Sklenar. He used the expressions "Kombucha mother tincture" and "Kombucha drops Dı". Dı in the homeopathic sense means that one part of medicinal preparation has been diluted with 9 parts of solvent. Dr. Sklenar prepared the drops himself and gave them to his patients. He obtained astonishing therapeutic results with them.

The drops obtained by pressing the culture are consequently not a fermented product, but are made from the kombucha culture itself. Obviously, there are other different component substances contained in the drops and in altered quantities.

How to make kombucha press extract

To make kombucha press extract use young kombucha mushrooms.

Method 1: Making a small amount: Take a garlic press and put some gauze in it. This is extremely laborious.

Method 2: An easier method to make mushroom press extract from surplus cultures is to cut the mushroom with scissors in to 2 up to 3cm thin strips. Squeeze these strips between your thumb and pointer finger out to the edges over a bowl or in a deep plate. A thin mushroom skin will remain which you can simply throw away.

Method 3: Use a blender shaft on already cut up pieces of mushroom and filter the slush through a fine gauze. (Methods 2 and 3 were shared with me by Kay Marcussen, Norderstedt).

Method 4: (for commercial use) The best way is to use an apothecary press which can be bought from a laboratory equipment retailer for about 300 euros. To make it non-perishable, mix the press extract 1:1 with 70% or 90% alcohol. I would not use alcohol as a preserving agent if you are using this privately and storing the concentrate in a fridge. The own acid content conserves the press extract. It is advisable only to prepare the amounts you would need for two weeks. It is generally recommended to take 15 drops in water three times a day.

According to Lück (1988), alcohol has a preservative effect in concentrations upwards of 18%, and according to Zettkin-Schaldach (1985, Vol. 1, p. 644), it has bactericidal properties (= it kills bacteria). Dittrich (1975, p. 74) mentions that yeast can continue to grow and ferment in 15% alcohol solution, but will be killed in a 25% alcohol solution. Professor Henneberg (1926, Handbuch der Gärungsbakteriologie, Vol. 1, p. 350) writes about experiments in which culture yeasts washed in 25% alcohol were killed in 39 minutes. Acetic bacteria were killed in 15 minutes by a 25% alcohol volume.

Because drops prepared according to the above-mentioned recipe with 70% alcohol consequently have a 35% alcohol content, the bacteria as well as the yeasts of the kombucha culture will accordingly be killed. The microorganisms of the kombucha culture can therefore hardly be the active substances of the drops. I suspect that the glucuronic acid contained in the mucilaginous matter, viz. the jelly-like part of the kombucha culture, is the significant substance.

Perhaps there's also something in the possibility of the polysaccharides coming into play here, which Dr. Schuitemaker (1988) wrote about and which have been obtained from fungi by scientific research in Japan and Korea. Schuitemaker writes that the polysaccharides in Ganoderma lucidum and japonicum (kombucha) have a special structure which in comparison to other medicinal plants possesses considerable biological activity. It is said to induce the immune system to seek identical structures on the surface of pathogenic bacteria, yeast plants and viruses. The author considers it very likely indeed "that the polysaccharides, for instance in kombucha, are capable of moderating this immunological response and of building up resistance to these diseases."

Independent of their active effect, a wide range of effectiveness in all kinds of illnesses is ascribed to kombucha drops. I know of naturopaths who report good results with these drops and who describe them as a concentrated form of kombucha therapy, which works more deeply and can accelerate the process of healing.

Candida and kombucha

Worried about Candida or other yeast infections? Don't be! Kombucha is a different kind of yeast-fungi. There are pathogen (harmful) and apathogen (harmless) yeasts. Kombucha is of the harmless kind.

Since kombucha is called a "mushroom" by many people, and a "fungus" by others, and since it is a yeast as well as a bacterial ferment, there are those who will automatically warn all candida albicans sufferers – those with chronic candiasis or any other kind of yeast infections – to stay away from kombucha.

However, this is not right. The Schizosacharomycodes, that is in the kombucha culture, is a yeast that is not in the family of candida, so it can be actually antagonistic to the troublesome yeast that infects so many people.

Kombucha is likely to be very beneficial for the following reason. Candida albicans is a yeast which competes with your bowel microflora and produces nothing in the way of benefit to the host organism. It occupies the body's defenses which have to be mobilized to oppose it. While this is going on your immune system can not effectively deal with other infections. Kombucha, on the other hand, is a community of microorganisms that do have a beneficial effect on the host, namely by producing glucuronic acid. The yeasts in kombucha compete with the candida yeasts and gradually replace them. They reproduce vegetative or by fission rather than by producing spores. This means that instead of having an enemy inside you, you have a friend.

In addition, you will also have some of the organisms which will colonize your gut somewhat and continue their good work. Provided that your batch is not contaminated with mold, there is nothing in kombucha that can harm you. It is true that certain people may have a sensitivity to it, but that can be elevated by reducing the dose. So that is about it. Nothing mystical! Nothing magical! and nothing harmful.

Prof. Rieth, Germany's leading expert in mycology based in Hamburg, confirmed to me: There is absolutely no risk in drinking kombucha as regards to yeast infections since the kombucha yeast is apathogenic. You can rely on his judgment based on careful research work. There are numerous scientific papers which prove, that there is no danger in preparing your own kombucha beverage. Prof. Rieth told me, there is very little knowledge of mycology (fungal diseases) even with doctors and many wrong allegations have been made.

The German "Bundesgesundheitsamt" (the top Public Health Office in Germany similar to the FDA in the USA) says: "Kombucha is not injurious to health." I hope that this is of value to some people who are worried by the fear and anxiety spread about KT by the tabloid media in particular.

Kombucha is no laughing matter for other mushrooms

The immune system can be strengthened by the kombucha beverage and this can counteract candida albicans. Normally, infections from naturally occurring fungi which may be taken into the body via the lungs or the bowel are no danger for an intact immune system. When we strengthen the body's immune defenses, we support our own bodily defenses against pathogenic fungi.

In addition, the probiotic lactic acid bacteria contained in kombucha can prevent and possibly heal candida infections. This was reported in the "New England Journal of Medicine": The lactobacilli are able to reduce considerably and prevent candida in laboratory cultures and in the human intestines. The Japanese doctor, Tsune-suke Tomoda administered leukemia patients bifido bacteria (lac-toacid creators) due to the unbearable suffering caused by chemo-therapy. There was a definite reduction of the yeast fungus flora in many of the patients and the fungus made them less susceptible to infections of the urinary tract and respiratory ducts.

This correlation helps us understand why many people report that kombucha has helped them to get their candida infections under control.

Should pregnant or nursing women drink kombucha?

There is still no definitive answer to this question. Pregnant and breast-feeding women should not drink kombucha as a precaution, unless they already drank kombucha for some months before their pregnancy. The reason is that glucuronic acid in kombucha binds own bodily metabolic poisons and environmental poisons foreign to the body and flushes them out. If you start drinking kombucha shortly before a pregnancy, the by-products could have a negative effect on the developing child. Mothers-to-be and breast-feeding mothers could also consider the following: kombucha beverages contain useful enzymes. These could, however, be too strong for the developing baby. Giving honey to babies less than one-year-old is also considered to be damaging because their metabolism cannot deal with it. This is the same reason for us to be reserved with our use of kombucha. Kombucha cleanses and supports the liver, the kidneys, the digestive system and purifies the body. A baby natural-ly does not need this.

Kombucha for children?

There is nothing damaging in kombucha. I would therefore not know any reason not to give kombucha to children. Kombucha is surely better for the little ones than sweet lemonade drinks. Naturally, they should start with small amounts. The adult dose should start at the age of about 18.

Kombucha tea made from herbal tea (decaffeinated) is preferable for children. Children like kombucha more when the acidy taste is somewhat milder. So make, for example, a special children's cocktail by mixing kombucha with mineral water, apple juice, raspberry syrup or black currant juice. It tastes good and is a great thirst quencher. By the way: kombucha is good for teenagers with acne

Is kombucha compatible with pharmaceuticals?

Taking a vast amount of different pharmaceutical medication can lead to side effects and interaction. Through this, the effect of a medication can be strengthened, weakened or even totally reversed. In addition to medication, nutrition and luxury foods can also interact with medicines. Examples include: the reciprocal strengthening effect of alcohol and tranquilizers, smoking leads to an accelerated break down and shorter benefits of many drugs, black tea reduces the absorption of many substances in the body, food intake reduces the absorption of many medicines, but, with fat-soluble components, can improve the absorption, grapefruit juice prevents the break down of many drugs.

Acidic drinks promote the resorption of many drugs. To be sure and to eliminate any interactions it is advisable not to drink any kind of acidic beverage two hours before or immediately after taking any medication, this includes kombucha.

What do you think
of kombucha in capsules?

Kombucha capsules are sold in pharmacies, chemists and on the internet. What makes me suspicious about them is that many companies seem to be riding on the good reputation of the kombucha beverage. I called a company selling kombucha capsules in a pharmacy and discovered that they contained the Japanese Kombu-Algae and not the tea mushroom. I had the same experience with a mail-order firm.

"Kombu" or also "Konbu" is the name for the brown alga (Laminaria Japonica or Saccharina Japonica, and probably other kinds), which are used as foodstuffs in Japan or in the production of tea. Despite the similarity of their names, the kombucha tea mushroom has nothing to do with this kelp-algae.

Nevertheless, capsules are offered for sale which actually do contain dried kombucha tea powder. A description from one company runs: One capsule contains 500mg of frozen dried kombucha tea. This equals the intake of half a glass of kombucha tea.

Recommendation: Inform yourself exactly about the ingredients if you turn to kombucha capsules. I personally prefer the kombucha beverage.

Can the kombucha culture be eaten?

If we accept the premise that the pressed juice contains substances which have a positive effect on our health, it is logical to assume that these substances are to be found in the culture itself, as the pressed juice is produced from nothing else but that. It is therefore entirely consistent if many people eat the culture directly. After all, there can be no other effective substances whether the culture is pressed, or crushed between the teeth.

There are scientists, however, who do not credit the culture as such with any useful properties, but only see the positive health effects in the metabolic products which have passed into the beverage.

The idea of eating the culture as well as drinking the fermented beverage was broached by Professor Lindner (1917/18). He suggests that to propagate the culture, one should peel off a thin layer from the old culture and use this for propagation purposes. Then he adds: "These young pieces of Bacterium xylinum can then be eaten on their own, but in any case this should be in addition to drinking the actual infusion. I suppose that this slippery, jelly-like masse passes easily through the intestines and helps to make them supple, particularly in cases of constipation."

I discovered that Wiechowski (1928) also tentatively approached the idea of eating the ready-formed cultures instead of drinking the fermented beverage, although in this case he was discussing various kinds of yogurt and kefir cultures. Without giving any definite opinion, he wrote the following in an article on the kombucha question:

"As is well known, Metchnikov believed that his bacteriological experiments furnished proof that the favorable, albeit more dietetic than therapeutic effects observed from the regular consumption of yogurt and kefir types of sour milk, are not due to the lactose that is produced by the action of the microorganisms concerned, but that it is the bacilli themselves which, when absorbed in large quantities through the consumption of this sour milk, influence the intestinal flora of man, in the sense of suppressing the Bacterium coli commune, the metabolic products of which Metchnikov considered were responsible for the appearance of certain symptoms of senility among other things and also for the appearance or the premature onset of arteriosclerosis. This opinion led Metchnikov to recommend the consumption of ready-prepared pure cultures of the schizomycete mixture also present in yogurt and kefir, as a suitable substitute for the regular consumption of sour milk of these types."

Part 6
Body, kitchen, cosmetics

Other methods of preparing kombucha

There are various methods of preparing kombucha which are in circulation, but, for the most part, vary from one another only very slightly. The diverse views on the quantity of sugar to be used, the length of fermentation time, etc., have already been mentioned in this book. I should like to add two more articles which are of interest and which present some new points of view.

The first article is by L. T. Danielova (1959). Her advice on how to prepare the beverage is given in a publication by the Ministry of Agriculture in the USSR, Institute of Zoological and Veterinary Science, Yerevan. In Danielova's work, particular consideration is given to the development of the antibacterial substances contained in kombucha. Tests were done to see which kind of nutrient solution would produce the most antibacterial substances. Extra nitrogen was added to the solution to increase the fermentation qualities of the yeasts. At the same time, it was established that the fermentation time is shortened and the activity accelerated when 0.3 % peptone is added. Besides feeding the solution with nitrogen, an infusion of apple was also added. The tests showed that, as a source of vitamins, the apple infusion had a beneficial effect on the active life of the culture.

Recipe by L. S. Danielova, Yerean (1959) for a kombucha beverage with high antibacterial effect

The author recommends the following nutrient solution, which proved to be particularly effective (quantities given are per liter of water):

- 2.5 grams tea
- 70 grams saccharose (= white sugar)
- 30 grams glucose (= dextrose)
- 3 grams peptone
- 15 grams apple tea
- hydrochloric or acetic acid to acidify the solution to pH 5.0-5.5.

Peptone is partly broken-down protein. Protein (e.g. the casein in milk) is predigested with an animal proteinase (pepsin), and the resulting peptideamino-acid mixture (= peptone)
added at 0.5–2.0 % to many bacteriological cultures.

First peptone and sugar are added to tap water. Then this solution is boiled, stirring continuously with a spatula. When completely dissolved the tea is boiled in this solution for 3-5 minutes, and then the solution is left to cool in the pan.

The apple tea is prepared separately, like this: leave dried apple rings to soak for a day and then boil for 5–10 minutes.

When the tea has cooled down to approx. 20–15 °C, it is acidified by the addition of hydrochloric or acetic acid to a pH value of 5.0–5.5, and is poured into a glass container. Then the required amount of apple tea is added.

The kombucha culture which is to be used to "inoculate" this new solution is cultivated beforehand in a medium made up in the same way and kept in a separate container of 1 to 3 liter capacity. On the third day, the culture with its fermentation liquid (10% of the larger amount of the new fermentation liquid) is transferred into the larger amount of the tea solution.

Danielova writes: "According to the results of our researches, the best growth of the culture takes place between 25 °C and 30 °C." She adds that the "seeding" must be carried out under conditions which are as sterile as possible, in order to avoid contaminating the culture with mold.

Marine alga – an account from Brazil, (author unknown)

The word "marine alga" is used. From the detailed description, this is the kombucha culture, which is often erroneously supposed to be partly composed of algae (in which case its classification among the lichens would be correct, as these are composed of algae and bacteria).

Prof. Xavier Filho (1985) of Paraiba University in Joao Pessoa, Brazil, writes about a culture commonly used in Brazil, called "auricularia delicata". As Prof. Filho told me, this culture is put into maté tea to make a medicinal beverage, and is also called "alga". I sent Prof. Filho a kombucha culture, and he confirmed that the Brazilian "alga" is identical to the kombucha culture.

I am publishing the Brazilian article because it contains some entirely new points of view and some suggestions for possible further applications, hitherto unknown to us over here. Wherever the word "alga" appears, read "kombucha". The Brazilian article contains some passages with which I cannot agree as far as kombucha is concerned (e.g. that the sugar can be left out, that the "alga" likes the sun, that peppermint or camomile tea can be used). When evaluating the advice, one should also certainly bear in mind that the climatic conditions of Brazil are completely different to those of Europe. Only a small part of the land lies in the temperate zone.

In tropical temperatures all fermentation processes take place with greater speed. Consequently, the fermentation times given in this article must be correspondingly lengthened for use under European conditions.

The original article from Brazil that I have here bears no indication of authorship or reference to a source. It is probably handed on in this form from one person to another. So as not to detract from the originality, I have left the article in its original form.

Brazilian instruction
"The marine alga" (identical to kombucha, just a different name). The marine alga is made of living cells, and these destroy the tired and sick cells in our body and also externally. Whoever cultivates such a marine alga has a real medicine chest in the house.

It cures the bronchial tubes, arthrosis, rheumatism, diabetes, leukemia, inflammation of the liver, bladder, uterus, ovaries, nerve problems, cleanses and restores the blood, cures haemo (N. B. probably means hemorrhoids), physical and mental lassitude, insomnia, respiratory problems, sore throat, wounds, even those which do not heal easily (then compresses are recommended), first-degree burns, anemia, regulates too high or too low blood pressure, impotence, and innumerable other diseases.

You lose weight, and in spite of that, your skin remains smooth, as only the surplus fat is burnt off. Cellulite will be avoided.

You can make an ointment to use for wrinkles. The skin will be soft as velvet.

For the hair: you rinse it with the tea of the alga, and it will be soft and shiny, also for hair gloss, it will grow back in.

To lose weight: 1 marine alga (identical with kombucha)
1 liter hot water
1 teaspoon black tea
2 dessertspoon sugar (allow to cool).

This amount 3 x is sufficient for 15 days. You prepare the tea, let it cool down, after that best to put in a glass container and lay the marine alga on top. Leave to infuse like this for 15 days. You cover the container with a light linen cloth, so that dust and dirt don't fall in. But never close with a lid, because the marine alga is a living organism and needs air to breathe.

After 15 days pour the tea into another container, and keep the tea like this in the fridge. After that, prepare fresh tea again. You drink a small glass of it 3 x a day before meals. This tea that has been left to infuse for 15 days ought to taste like a dry white wine. Young algae have a rather sharper taste.

The important thing is that during the time when you are losing weight, at the same time you will also be healed of a disease you maybe didn't even have any idea you had, and you will be well. It takes a while until you lose weight, but after that, there's no stopping it. When you have reached your weight, don't throw the marine alga away, but just leave it to infuse for a few days. You can even leave out the sugar, as the marine alga doesn't absorb all of the sugar in a few days. The sugar is only important for losing weight.

When you have reached your weight, let the tea infuse for only 10-8 or even 6 days, and then drink also 3 x a day after meals. But you must learn how to handle the marina alga yourself. After that, you can even drink a glass day after day, as a refreshment.

To lose weight quicker, always use an older marine alga, as it takes a bit longer when you use a young one; the older the better, whether you are using it so slim or as a cure. The important thing about it is, you lose weight and nevertheless have no problems with your health, as the marine alga does you only good.

If you have serious problems with cellulite, then massage the place with the tea and let it dry.

A marine alga like this does not die so easily; even if it is cut in pieces, it carries on reproducing itself. For when you notice a piece of the marine alga detaching itself, that is another young offshoot. Make some more tea at once, and put the young alga in it so that it can start growing again.

Let the young marine alga infuse for only 6 days, then it can even be given to children to drink each day. When you exchange the marine alga, you should wash it up (off) carefully. The marine alga also likes the sun; now and then it can be left open. Only be careful about flies and dust.

For illnesses:

If you are ill but do not want to lose weight, let the tea infuse for only 10, 9 or 8 days. Remember, you must learn how to handle the marine alga yourself.

So you are drinking it then 3 x a day before meals, for 3 months, even if you sometimes let it infuse for 15 days, only after that you should begin with fewer days. For the tea is not just meant for losing weight; it also purifies poisons, impurities in the organism, in the blood. If you have drunk the tea and experience any kind of reactions during the first days, no need to get agitated, it will be all right again, only don't stop drinking the tea, for it will restore a feeling of well-being and youth.

Even pregnant women should drink the tea; they can thereby avoid poisons of any sort from forming in the cells.

Wrinkles can be softened too. For facial wrinkles a cream is made from a large marine alga. It is chopped up fine in an electric mixer, mixed with a little of the prepared tea, after that kept in the fridge in an open container. The cream is used like a face mask; leave to work in for an hour. For this purpose, you should lie down and shut your eyes, but don't go to sleep; this is the best way for the cram to take effect. The notorious crow's-feet around the eyes disappear in a month. Anyone with serious skin problems should use this cream every day; thereafter wash off with cold water, then dab the face with a swab of cotton wool dipped in tea, and leave to dry. Even if you don't have any cream yet, you can wash your face with the tea in the morning and in the evening before going to bed. After that you can continue to use a day-cream or make-up. Even unsightly blemishes on the skin disappear.

Hair: wash and rinse hair as usual, then with the marine alga tea as the final rinse. Helps with hair loss too.

Have no doubts or fears about drinking this marine alga tea. It is a natural product and cannot do any harm.

If you do not want to lose weight, you could also make the tea from peppermint, camomile, or other sorts for a change. Entirely according to your taste.

Good luck with your marine alga. And don't forget: it is a living organism, take care of it.

Note: the above is no recommendation of mine, but comes from Brazil. It is published for documentary purposes only, to show how the kombucha culture is regarded in other parts of the world. Perhaps it contains some suggestions, however, which could be pursued further.

Refreshing drinks with kombucha

There are numerous variations for preparing delicious mixed drinks with kombucha. Here are a few for some inspiration.

Refreshing drink with herbs:
1 liter apple juice
1 liter ice tea (Lemon)
1 liter kombucha (sour, i.e. long fermentation period)
1 Bunch of fresh, seasonal herbs e.g. peppermint, elderberry blossom.
English mint, sweet balm, borage, daisies etc.
1 lemon, cut in slices
Ice cubes (perhaps with some decorative blossom frozen in them)
1–2 Bottle of fizzy water
Throw in a handful of herbs and leave them in the beverage (without the fizzy water) for 2 to 3 hours and leave to cool. Squeeze the herbs thoroughly before removing them. Add ice cubes and lemons and serve. Add the fizzy water (⅓ fizzy water to 2/3 herbal kombucha) and drink up. Tip: This drink changes its taste at will, but, is always delicious and refreshing, a little bit like the Austrian non-alcohol herbal lemonade, Almdudler.

Refreshing drink with elderberry juice
1.5 liter of kombucha
0.2 liter home made elderberry juice
1 knife tip of vitamin C (ascorbic acid)
Glucose (perhaps to sweeten afterwards)
1 liter fizzy water
Ice cubes

This beverage has a very original taste, but, is also deliciously thirst-quenching. Once you have started drinking it, you can't stop.

Bubbly Kombucha Cocktails
Gerd Käfer gave me the following recipes (Feinkost-Käfer, Munich) in December 2000 with the personal permission to publish them in my book. Thank you Mr Käfer!

"Gemüsekäfer/Vegetable Beetle"(non-alcoholic)
0.1 liter carrot juice, 0.1 liter freshly squeezed orange juice, 0.1 liter kombucha plus one dash of tonic water on ice and serve in a long-drink glass. Take a long "macaroni" as a straw and a small carrot as garnish.

"Fit and fun" (non-alcoholic)
0.1 liter currant juice, 0.1 liter mineral water and 0.1 liter kombucha served in a long-drink glass

"Shape it" (non-alcoholic)
Squeeze 2 Oranges, 1 large Grapefruit and 1 lemon fill up with 0.1 liter kombucha.

Dessert: Kombucha Sorbet
0.1 liter chilled kombucha in a champagne cup and pour over a scoop of fruit ice-cream, garnished with fresh fruit and some aniseed biscuits. Don't forget your spoon and straw.

Kombucha Soup

Take: ½ liter kombucha beverage, 4 onions, butter, salt, pepper, curcuma, 1 teaspoon vegetable stock, 1 tablespoon of grated hard cheese.

Peel the onions and cut into small pieces, flavour with salt, pepper and curcuma and fried to golden yellow in butter. Pour in the kombucha, the vegetable stock and then melt the cheese in the soup. The delicious kombucha soup is ready! Now enjoy it!

Preparation time: approx 15 minutes

Many thanks to Dietmar Fischer, Saarbrücken, who gave me this recipe.

Kombucha Bread

Frau E. B. from F. in Switzerland sent me the following letter:
Dear Mr Frank, I have just taken my kombucha bread out of the oven and am enjoying its wonderfully delicious aroma. Each time I smelt the scent of yeast as I emptied the tea beverage I had made, I wondered if I should drink yeast or bake it. As I love experiments, I baked it. The result is more than satisfying. Here is my recipe considered as the basis for further experimentation:

750 grams whole meal flour (not too heavy), 1 tablespoon salt, 50 ml bottom yeast (use more depending on flour), dissolved in 10 day fermented kombucha. 450 ml water (lukewarm). For sour bread, a dash of kombucha vinegar if desired.

Knead before it rises, afterwards shape. Allow the dough to rise 3 to 4 hours in warmth. Form a round loaf, cut into it and leave to rise again. Then bake at 200 °C (40 minutes)

Kombucha vinegar

Lakowitz (1928) wrote in the Apotheker-Zeitung (Pharmaceutical Times) that if the kombucha culture is allowed to work for a longer period of time, "an aromatic liquid just like vinegar" is obtained, "which can be put to excellent use as vinegar and is preferable to commercially available spirit vinegar because it tastes milder – and is cheaper than the usual vinegar." And Henneberg (1928) also mentions that "any tea kvass that has accidentally gone too sour can be used as table vinegar."

So it's not disastrous if you sometimes have to leave the fermented beverage for longer than usual, e.g. if you go away for a long holiday.

The resultant vinegar is vaguely reminiscent in taste to cider vinegar, and can be used for cooking, to make salad dressing, and in other dishes. It should, however, rather not be used to preserve food, e.g. pickling gherkins, because it is still biologically "active" and is not sterilized.

Kombucha for your pet

The first research into the use of the household remedy, kombucha, for veterinary use was in Russia in 1947. The results showed that kombucha is also beneficial to animals. The dosage must be adapted to the size and weight of the animal. A horse needs more than a terrier. A herbivore has a different digestive system to a carnivore. Try giving your animal kombucha gradually to see if it agrees with it.

Methods of administering:
- You could add some kombucha to the drinking water depending on the size of the animal, for example.

- Feed them some bread soaked in some kombucha. Start with small rations so that your pet gradually gets used to the taste.

- If you feed your animal with pellets, you can soak them in kombucha.

- Mix some kombucha beverage or pureed kombucha mushroom in the animal food.

- For treating skin problems, dab the affected area with a ball of cotton wool soaked in kombucha.

Part 7

Calories and alcohol

How many calories does the beverage contain?

I have not succeeded in finding anyone who would commit themselves unequivocally to stating how many calories or kilojoules there are in kombucha. This of course is not possible, for the simple reason that these values depend on the acidity level, which varies from case to case. Even those who produce ready-made kombucha, who must surely strive to achieve a degree of acidity that is as constant as possible, could give me no data.

I have therefore tried to draw up a few theories of my own. These however are not definitive, as they are not tested to laboratory standards.

White sugar has a calorific value of 1650 kJ = 394 kcal. If 70 grams/liter is used to make kombucha, one would get 1155 kJ = 276 kcal.

Through the fermentation process, part of the sugar is used up. The residual sugar content of the completed beverage is determined by the degree of fermentation, which in turn is dependent on various factors. Because the beverage for reasons of taste is generally not left to ferment completely, a proportion of residual sugar remains – as it does with wine.

If we suppose a residual sugar content of 30 g/l, this means 495 kJ = 118 kcal. A residual sugar content of 20 g/l works out at 330 kJ = 79 kcal.

With a correspondingly longer fermentation period, which naturally must be paid for by concessions to one's taste-buds, an even lower calorific value can be reached.

When considering calorific figures, one must also take into account the fact that these may be by the metabolic processes activated by the beverage.

Kombucha helps to lose weight

Kombucha is the ideal partner for losing weight. The fermented beverage can speed up the most lethargic of metabolisms and help regulate digestion. There is far better bowel movement and the body is purified. At the same time the beverage regenerates your intestinal flora, digestive tract and whole organism. Kombucha awakens your spirits and boosts the digestive system. Kombucha can't reduce your weight if you generally eat too much. And reducing fat is certainly not to be achieved with kombucha. Kombucha can, however, be a good support to use due to its appetite reducing effect.

Alcohol content of kombucha

A small amount of alcohol is contained in the fermented kombucha beverage. The formation of alcohol depends largely on the constituent yeasts in the culture, the fermentation temperature, the amount of sugar use, and other factors. Reiss (1987), who used 50 grams of sugar per liter of tea, found an alcohol content of 0.1 % after 14 days and 0.35 % after 21 days. Löwenheim (1927), who used the extremely high amount of 125 grams of sugar per liter of tea, found 0.91 % alcohol after 7 days, 1.43 % after 10 days, and 2.18 % after 15 days. In the meantime, however, the degree of acidity had risen so high in Löwenheim's beverage that it had become undrinkable ("very sour indeed; drew my cheeks together"). Harms (1927) gives an average alcohol content of 1% in a pleasant tasting beverage.

A normal, home-made preparation should probably reach an average alcohol content of around 0.5 % or slightly higher. This is as much as you get in so-called alcohol-free beer. Normal beer contains about ten times as much percentage of alcohol (3-8%). 0.5 % alcohol is also found in many fruit juices, by the way, and even in some sorts of white bread. This slight amount of alcohol is normally harmless. For alcoholics, however, it means "hands off kombucha!" The Blue Cross in Wuppertal confirmed my query.

Professor Rainer Tölle from the Psychiatry Clinic of Münster University has also recently warned rehabilitated alcoholics in particular against drinking so-called alcohol-free beer and fruit juices. Because of their high sensitivity to the psychological and physiological effects of alcohol, even such small amounts can still be dangerous for them. This warning can be correspondingly transferred to the similar amount of alcohol contained in kombucha.

"test" magazine (No. 1/89) gives a similar assessment of wine from which the alcohol content has been removed; it still contains up to 0.5 % per cent by volume alcohol, viz. about as much as kombucha. "From a quite sober and purely medical point of view, this beverage with its mini percent would be suitable even for alcoholics at risk, children or sick people. However, one cannot overestimate the psychological factor, which is exactly what could lead to the risk of danger, particularly for dried out alcoholics."

Part 8

Sugar and honey

Sugar in kombucha

The "problem"

Kombucha drinkers are generally health-conscious people who think about what they are eating and drinking. They know that with regard to sugar in the whole field of wholefood – irrespective of a variety of other often mutually contradictory views about nutrition – everyone is agreed that the use of refined white sugar should in principle be disapproved of.

Dr. Schnitzer (1982) and Dr. Bruker (1981), well-known German nutrition experts, stress emphatically that there is absolutely no need for any refined sugar in the human organism, and that "the fate or a person's physical condition depends in large measure upon what they decide their attitude is towards the substance sugar" (Bruker, Foreword to Binder and Wahler, 1987). Saying "No" to sugar is the most important step towards healthy nutrition.

The use of sugar in the preparation of Kombucha therefore worries many people and gives them a guilty conscience. For this reason, I think it would be useful to examine the sugar question in rather more detail.

A little about "sugar chemistry"

In chemistry, the sugars, besides containing starch, glycogen and cellulose and their derivatives, are counted as carbohydrates. Carbohydrates, including sugar, consist of the elements carbon (C), hydrogen (H), and oxygen (O), which can be seen for example in the formula for glucose: $C_6H_{12}O_6$. Carbohydrates are a product of assimilation by plants. Assimilation denotes the process of metabolism and energy production by which plants by the supply of energy gradually convert extraneous substances which they have absorbed, into fluids and tissues identical with their own.

Sugar can be divided into two big groups:
1. Simple sugars or monosaccharides.
2. Compound sugars, which are produced by dehydration from monosaccharide units. Compound sugars can again be divided into:
a) Oligosaccharides, which consist of two to ten units
b) Polysaccharides, which form chains out of many monosaccharides.

In the oligosaccharide group, it is the disaccharides (2 monosaccharide residues linked together) which are of the greatest biological importance. They are combinations of two simple sugar molecules. So, for example, in white household sugar (saccharose) one molecule of glucose is combined with one molecule of fructose. In the disaccharide lactose, one molecule each of glucose and galactose have combined. In maltose, two molecules of glucose have combined.

Chemists represent our normal white sugar thus:

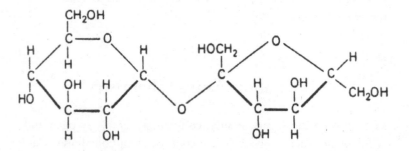

On the right, the five-cornered ring of fructose can be seen and, on the left, the six-cornered ring of glucose. In the middle the linking atom of oxygen can be seen. This link is easily divisible.

Through the influence of enzymes or acids, disaccharide – i.e. our household sugar – can decompose into two parts: into the monosaccharides (simple sugar) glucose and fructose.

The chemical splitting of chemical links by the agency of water, dilute acids or enzymes is called hydrolysis. By this hydrolysis, the originally right-hand rotating (dextrogyral) saccharose will be decomposed into a left-hand rotating (levogyral) mixture of equal parts of D-glucose and D-fructose. Because of this alteration in the direction of rotation, the hydrolysis of saccharose is also referred to as inversion.

This process of inversion, by the way, also takes place in the human digestive system. The digestive enzymes of the small intestine and the pancreas break down the large molecule of granulated sugar (saccharose) in the digestive organs into two smaller molecules: a glucose molecule and a fructose molecule. The system can digest glucose and fructose better than saccharose. Glucose is absorbed directly into the blood and converted into living matter by the process called metabolism.

Processes of building up, breaking down, and conversion are going on all the time in the body. During the course of this, glucose is stored in the system in the storage form of glycogen, as a reserve for periods of low energy. Glycogen is found above all in the liver and in the muscle cells. Once the limited storage space is full, the rest is converted into fat.

It is an established fact that the basic nutrient of every cell is sugar. A human being requires natural sugar as it is found in unaltered foodstuffs, e.g. fruit, vegetables, cereals, etc. (Bruker and Gutjahr, 1982).

Sugar is without doubt the chief energy provider for a human. However, we don't need to use refined sugar for that purpose. The human organism is much better able to produce sugar (glucose, blood-sugar) from other carbohydrates. The starch contained above all in cereals and potatoes is converted into blood-sugar and thus into energy, by a complicated biochemical process.

Aids towards the breakdown and utilization of substances are the enzymes, vitamins and minerals which the body must be given in adequate amounts each day. Vitamin B1 is one of these. It is needed by the metabolism for the utilization of sugar. There is sufficient vitamin B1 in grain, in coarse-ground whole-meal bread and in potatoes to convert the carbohydrates contained in these foodstuffs. Refined white sugar, however, is lacking in vitamin B1. Thus refined sugar can indirectly rob the system of vitamin B1, as it needs it for the process of conversion.

Why is white sugar recommended for the preparation of kombucha?

What do the above remarks mean in connection with kombucha? We have seen that every cell requires sugar. The human organism is able to produce the requisite blood-sugar from other carbohydrates. It is therefore not dependent on refined sugar in order to do this.

The kombucha culture, however, is dependent on the supply of sugar, because it cannot produce it itself in sufficient quantities on its own. It has to be supplied with sugar in the nutrient solution.

Sugar plays an important part in the metabolism of the kombucha culture, during the feeding, breathing and fermentation of the microorganisms. The kombucha culture can only accomplish as much the energy it is supplied with. The metabolic processes, including the process of conversion of energy connected with them, are essential for all organisms. Therefore sugar is absolutely essential in the making of kombucha.

Hence, sugar is not added to kombucha to make the beverage taste sweeter, but to form a good nutrient solution for the culture. The culture feeds on the sugar and draws energy from it, as well as from the minerals and the nitrogen which have passed into the liquid from the tea leaves, energy which is needed for its metabolic activity while it makes the various component parts of the kombucha beverage, grows, and forms offshoots.

Let's hear what Prof. Henneberg (1926b, p.7) has to say:
"The yeast cells must absorb nutrients to build up their cell body, replenish substances eliminated through the continually ongoing process of metabolism, and obtain the necessary energy to live. This latter is obtained by respiration (oxidation) and fermentation. Sugar is used for nutrition (assimilation) as well as for respiration and most of all for fermentation. Glucose is the best for almost all kinds of yeasts; other kinds of sugar can only be fermented or used as nutrient by isolated types of yeast. Types of sugar which are fermentable do not need to be, at the same time, assimilable, and conversely, those which are assimilable do not have to fermentable."

During the fermentation period of kombucha (we will call the process "fermentation" for the sake of simplicity, although what takes place is not just fermentation in the strictest sense of the word) various metabolic processes take place within the tea solution. So, for example, assimilation processes take place during the growth of yeast cells and bacteria, as has already been mentioned. At the same time, dissimilation processes are also taking place. The balance between assimilation and dissimilation ensure that things are constantly circulating in Nature ("The law of conservation of energy").

Dissimilation is the process of metabolism and formation of energy by which organic matter is more or less broken down by the release of energy into other end products. Dissimilation can take place as respiration (biological oxidation) or as fermentation.

Biological oxidation does not take place directly, but by a chain of several processes of reduction and oxidation which are initiated (catalyzed) by enzymes (respiration chain).

If the processes of dissimilation take place when oxygen is present (= aerobic breakdown), this is called **r**espiration; if they take place without oxygen, this is called **fermentation** (= anaerobic breakdown). However, the aerobic breakdown of ethanol in acetic acid ("acetic acid fermentation") or of glucose in citric acid is also designated as fermentation. In both kinds of dissimilation, the energy hereby obtained is used for numerous vital functions or processes of synthesis.

Alcoholic fermentation means that when there is insufficient atmospheric oxygen, the yeast plants break down the sugar into ethyl alcohol and carbon dioxide (breakdown without atmospheric oxygen, intramolecular breakdown or fermentation). If, however, free oxygen is available for the yeast cells, then they can, like other plants, burn the sugar up completely (respiration of oxygen, aerobic breakdown). Thus, they have been made capable of both kind of dissimilation. (From Lindner, 1967, p. 96, 97, 62).

The yeast plants in the kombucha culture bring about the development of alcohol and carbon or carbonic acid by intermediate stages from the component parts of the sugar in the nutrient substratum. Besides alcohol and carbon, further numerous organic acids are formed by the effect of the yeasts. The alcohol is in turn transformed by biochemical oxidation into acetic acid and other acids by the action of Bacterium xylinum and other bacteria.

According to Heimann (1976, p. 491), we should speak "of **dehydration** rather than of oxidation, as it is not oxygen which is activated by the enzymes of the bacteria, the alcohol dehydratases, but hydrogen."

Various processes of fermentation and respiration occur during the preparation of kombucha. These are extremely complicated processes which happen gradually in a chain of consecutive and simultaneous reactions. Processes involving the binding and releasing of energy occur which stand in reciprocal relation to one another. Assimilation and dissimilation are bound up with one another in this, and overlap. During the course of these biological forms of movement of matter, sugar is broken down and transformed into acids, vitamins, carbon dioxide, antibiotic substances, water, etc. At the same time, sugar serves as a source of energy for the growth and propagation of the kombucha culture.

For these reasons, the sugar in the kombucha beverage is not harmful – precisely because by the end of the fermentation proceed it will have been transformed (to a large extent at least) into another form of energy. The starting sugar, through the action of the kombucha culture, may be almost completely used up if the process of fermentation is not prematurely broken off.

This is confirmed by Dr. Bruker (1986), who otherwise sees red whenever sugar is mentioned. In answer to a reader's query, he pointed out that the transformation of the sugar substances in kombucha corresponds to the processes of fermentation by microbes during the production of curdled milk, kefir, yogurt, etc. After 10 days, the starting sugar has long since been fermented. However, Dr. Bruker limits this opinion to the effect that it is only valid if one starts the beverage off oneself (with honey) and leaves it sufficiently long to ferment. Then the sugar will be completely transformed, and the beverage tastes correspondingly tart. The beverages to be found on the market, however, taste so very sweet that you can tell from the taste alone that they contain relatively high amounts of refined sugar, which may be detrimental to diabetics, those with easily upset stomachs and bowels, cancer patients, etc.

Sugar is transformed
The breakdown of sugar is confirmed by the results of the analyses by Dr. Jürgen Reiss (1987). He published the result of his analyses under the title "The kombucha culture and its metabolic products" in the "Deutsche Lebensmittelrundschau" (German Food Review) No. 9/1987, and reports: "Through the action of the yeasts which splits the cane sugar, sufficient glucose is released to become oxidized into gluconic acid by means of Bacterium gluconicum (p. 287).

Cane sugar is hydrolyzed by means of the enzymes of the yeasts, which split the saccharose, and by acetic acid bacteria. This is manifested by a rapid rise in the glucose concentration measured in the tea, from the 5th to the 9th day. Now begins a marked increase in the metabolic processes which break down the glucose, and these lead to a swift decrease in the glucose content. Parallel to this, there is an increased concentration of ethanol and organic acids as products of metabolism. Diagrammatic representation (see p. 79 of this book) shows clearly an increase in the formation of lactic acid, gluconic acid and ethanol within 6 to 12 days after fermentation has begun. An expression of the increase in the formation of acids is a decrease in the pH value. Around the 17th day, the reserves of glucose are nearly exhausted, and then the measured metabolic products have already reached their maximal value" (p. 289).

In another experiment, which was conducted by Dinslage and Ludorff (1927), the component parts of sugar in kombucha were likewise examined. The result: "The original tea infusion, to which 10 grams of saccharose per 100 ml had been added, contained only 3.25 grams of this latter after some 14 days. Inversion and fermentation had used up the 6.75 grams."

Hermann (1928) reaches the following results concerning the classification of sugar before and after acidification by the kombucha culture: "On the 3rd of June a solution of tea and cane sugar with a saccharose content of 11.7 % was inoculated. On the 11th of July the saccharose content amounted to 3.6 %. From 11.7 grams of cane sugar, 8.1 grams were transformed into the following combinations: 2.69 grams gluconic acid, 1.90 grams acetic acid, 3.42 grams invert sugar."

Hermann writes that under favorable conditions, up to 80% of the weight of the glucose available in 10% solution can be transformed into gluconic acid (p. 180). In another experiment, Hermann found that after 5 weeks' fermentation time, 11% of the original glucose content was still available (p. 185).

These reports and results prove unequivocally:

1. Sugar is required for the preparation of kombucha.

2. It is however to a large extent transformed.

At most one could still argue about two questions, which will be discussed in the next sections:

1. How much sugar should be used?

2. What sort of sugar should be used?

How much sugar should one use?

Many authors seem to consider precise rules about the quantity of sugar to be quite unimportant. So, for example, the directions issued by the Chemical and Bacteriological Laboratory of the Pure Yeast Culture Institute at Kitzingen am Main, which were quoted by Arauner (1929), say that one should sugar the tea "to taste."

In most of the directions and research articles, however, we find more or less exact recommendations about the amount of sugar to be used. Nevertheless, the details about the weight diverge from one another quite considerably at times.

I found the smallest quantity in an answer to a reader's letter in "Naturarzt" (Naturopath 12/88), in which Dr. Abele (1988) advises a diabetic to use only 40 grams of sugar per liter of tea.

Prof. W. Henneberg (1926 b) recommends 50 grams of sugar per liter of nutrient solution.

The recommendation to use 50 grams is found in other authors as well. To my way of thinking, however, such small amounts should only be used when the liquid is going to be left to ferment for a particularly short time. Then a higher concentration would have no sense, as larger amounts will not be used up in a shorter working time.

I found the maximum quantity of sugar, as mentioned in the literature on it, in Harms (1927), though in my opinion this is definitely set too high. Dr. Harms of Berlin mentions that he obtained directions from a private source on how to make kombucha, according to which one should use 1½ lbs. per 4 liters of water. Converted to 1 liter, this is 187.5 grams.

Yet, most authors mention weights of about 100 grams.

Don't let the mushroom get hungry

I personally believe that the correct weight recommendation is "70 to 100 grams" of sugar. For my own family kombucha, I tend to use around 70 grams. One should not, however, put in less than 70 grams, otherwise the culture goes without food and cannot work properly.

When aiming for a small amount of residual sugar, I don't think it's so very important to use a small amount of starting sugar, but it's vital to leave the beverage to ferment for long enough. If you're not just going to drink the beverage on account of its pleasant taste, viz. for reasons of pleasure, but also value the wholesome metabolic products, then the question arises whether there's really any advantage in using a small amount of sugar. For when less sugar is available in the nutrient solution for the culture, it will be able to develop fewer metabolic products during the process of fermentation, which is what matters to us.

The Soviet scientists, G. A. Sakaryan and L. T. Danielova (1948) also came to this conclusion. Through their series of experiments, they established that the effectiveness of the kombucha beverage is connected to the glucose content of the nutrient solution. With a 10% glucose content (100 grams per 1 liter of tea) the activity of the infusion is double what it is with a 5% content.

A selection of four variants

It would seem to only make sense then to use less starting sugar when the fermentation process is going to be prematurely broken off. With less starting sugar, we also get a lower content of the residual sugar, which so many people find undesirable. If, however, we leave the beverage to ferment thoroughly, the logical chain of thought can only look like this:

1. Small amount of starting sugar + short period of fermentation = little energy = few metabolic products + little residual sugar
2. Small amount of starting sugar + long period of fermentation = little energy = few metabolic products + almost no residual sugar
3. Adequate starting sugar + short period of fermentation = a lot of energy = relatively few metabolic products + almost no residual-sugar
4. Adequate starting sugar + long period of fermentation = a lot of energy = a lot of metabolic products + little residual sugar (+ sour taste)

Theoretically, we arrive at the same residual sugar content, whether we use less sugar and leave it to ferment for a shorter period, or whether we use more sugar and leave it to ferment for longer. The second variant seems to me to be the more sensible, on account of the higher content in metabolic products. Another point to consider is naturally the question of what it tastes like. In longer fermented tea with more starting sugar, more acids will be formed through conversion. Concerning the acid content, other opinions could naturally come into play ("acid/alkali problem"). Depending on how high each person rates the individual factors, they will decide on one of the 4 formulas listed above.

Are there alternatives to white sugar?

Synthetic sweetener
Synthetic sweeteners such as saccharin and cyclamate bear no relationship whatsoever to sugar. They provide no energy, but only a sweet taste. Under no circumstances can they be used to make kombucha.

Sugar substitutes
Sugar substitutes are various sugar alcohols (polyole): sorbit (E 420), isomalt (E 953), mannitol (E 421), maltit (E 965), maltitol syrup (E 965), lactit (E 966) and xylitol (E 967). These are sweet tasting carbohydrates, which have less influence on the blood sugar level than household sugar.

Sugar substitutes can not be fermented. They are therefore not suitable for making kombucha. They can be used individually, like sweeteners, to give the fermented kombucha tea a sweeter taste but not for the fermentation process.

Brown sugar

There is often a great deal of ignorance concerning brown sugar which is offered for sale in food stores and health food shops. Not all sugar which is of a brown color is more nutritious than white sugar.

There are roughly speaking two sorts of brown sugar:

1. Brown sugar which is manufactured from refined white sugar, and which gets its brownish color and relatively poor flavor from the addition of molasses or caramel. This brown sugar is not much different from white sugar expect in color. It consists of up to 96% refined sugar to which only 3-4% molasses has been added. This brown sugar is often erroneously regarded as being particularly nutritious, but it has, like white sugar, virtually no vital elements except for a minute portion of trace elements in the molasses residue.

2. Unrefined brown sugar which is extracted directly from the sugar cane. This sugar, which can be called "raw cane sugar", has a brown color and a strong flavor, due to the way it is manufactured. Under raw sugar we can again differentiate two sorts:

a) Raw cane sugar which is actually destined for the manufacture or refined white sugar. It is manufactured from sugar cane in the countries of origin by a process which is little concerned about cleanliness, and brought to Europe in great shiploads for further processing. A limited amount of this sugar is not processed into white sugar, but is cleaned of outward impurities with superheated steam and then sold as pure can cane sugar.

b) The better quality pure cane sugar is already processed into the finished product in the country of origin. During the manufacturing process, importance is attached to cleanliness right from the start. A subsequent steambath is not required. With the sugar, there are further possibilities of differentiation through a variety of manufacturing processes which result in differing values of the constituent elements and in products with differing characteristics.

Whole cane sugar

As a healthy alternative to white sugar, only cane sugar really comes into consideration, as mentioned in the previous paragraph under 2 b). Various designations are used for cane sugar of this kind: whole cane sugar, dried sugarcane juice, natural sugar, etc. As far as the basic meaning is concerned, "raw sugar" should really be equivalent to "whole sugar". In actual fact, however, "raw sugar" is mostly equated with the concept "brown sugar", and this has long been traditional. In order to avoid misunderstanding, I should therefore like to use the term "whole cane sugar".

In the magazine "Wissenschaft in der UdSSR" (Science in the USSR – No. 6/8), Dr. Brechmann and Dr. Grinewitsch develop a method by which the various groups of basic and luxury foods are evaluated according to the structural information contained within them. They call the information which reflects the measure of the diversity and complexity of the inner structure, absolute or structural information. With the help of computers, the range of structural information was comprised in "bits" (the measure for a unit of information) for a range of medicinal and basic foodstuffs with varying degrees of refinement, and subsequently divided into 4 groups:

o group	1st group	2nd group	3rd group
o–1 bit	1,1–10 bits	10,1–99 bits	100 and more bits

Examples (excerpt):

caffeine	– – –	tea, coffee	– – –
white sugar	golden sugar	sweet fruit, honey	– – –
vitamins	polyvitamins	berries, fruit, vegetables, herbs and spices	vegetable salad, stewed fruit

According to this system, tea, for example, is to be classified higher than pure caffeine because it contains other information as well. It is much the same thing with the sugar group. The authors have this to say about it: "In contrast to this (viz. refined sugar), raw golden sugar is to be considerably more recommended, as it possesses a range of useful qualities."

Rather less scientifically expressed, you could thus say: If you have to use sugar, then use whole cane sugar, because it contains more positive "structural information" (vitamins, mineral salts, trace elements, amino acids, etc.), which partly counterbalance the negative structural information.

This view, however, would not be unanimously supported in this form by all advocates of a healthy way of life. Dr. Bruker, for example, rejects all kinds of manufactured sugar, including even "whole cane sugar preparations."

Evaluation of unrefined cane sugar in the preparation of kombucha

On account of the sometimes really positive reports about unrefined cane sugar, it became obvious to me that unrefined cane sugar should be preferable for the preparation of kombucha, because of its minerals and other constituent elements. I even managed to lay my hands on recipes in which "Sucanat" (100% whole cane sugar) is recommended.

I therefore started off several fermentation processes using Sucanat. The result was a very different beverage indeed from kombucha made with refined white sugar. Instead of the relatively clear, clean and pleasant tasting tea, I got a rather cloudy, dark brown fluid that looked rather unappetizing and was unappealing to taste. The beverage tasted slightly less acidic than the nutrient solution fermented with refined white sugar. The lower acid content was confirmed by measuring the pH value. Apart from that, the beverage developed hardly any carbonic acid, even after a few days of secondary fermentation in the bottle, although a thicker (yeast?) sediment built up at the bottom. The strong malty flavor of the Sucanat still came through very distinctly. I suppose that the substances (possibly also the natural "impurities", viz. bits of sugar cane) contained in the concentrated sugar cane juice hand inhibited the development of the microorganisms in the kombucha culture and had not supplied it with sufficient energy. Several people, who had also tried experimenting with Sucanat, wrote to me saying that they had arrived at similar fermentation results which were not wholly satisfactory.

Herr Erich Rasche of Friesenheim was so kind as to thoroughly examine the difference between Kombucha made with refined white sugar and kombucha made with Sucanat, and to measure it by means of bio-electronics, using the Vincent method (BE). Erich Rasche is an expert in the field of BE and together with Dr. Morell has written a few publications on this subject. The biological terrain of liquids can be physically measured by means of BE. Using the physical units of measurement pH (acid/alkali value), rH_2 (electron potential) and r (specific resistance, mineral content), conclusions can be drawn abut the substances which are beneficial to the organism.

Herr Rasche sent me the following results of the measurement:

Kombucha I ("Sucanat" whole cane sugar):

pH = 3.76, rH_2 = 21.5, r = 429.

The measurement r = 429 indicates a large amount of minerals in a good terrain.

Kombucha II (white sugar):

pH = 2.92, rH_2 = 24.1, r = 1740.

The measurement r = 1740 ohms shows that no minerals are present in the sugar.

Generally speaking: should a foodstuff provide **energy**, it should, if at all possible, be from the terrain in the 1st zone (Note: in bio-electronics, the liquid medium is divided into 4 zones), acid-reduced, i.e. producing many protons and many electrons. In addition, as many assimilable minerals as possible (small r unit of measurement).

If I wanted an **energy-provider**, I would use sample I (**kombucha made with Sucanat**).

If I wanted an **immune stimulation agent**, I would use sample II (**Kombucha made with white sugar**).

As concerns kombucha, I understand that the beverage is intended to improve the immune system of man and beast.

Whether one can now compare the two samples with one another depends solely on whether the conditions were the same for both samples. I mean, the same length of fermentation time, the same amount of white sugar or Sucanat, and above all, water of the same quality."

Herr Rasche's measurement result can naturally only relate to the two samples I sent him. I should point out that both beverages had been produced under the same conditions (8 days' fermentation, 80 g/l refined white sugar or Sucanat unrefined whole can sugar respectively), with the same Birkenfeld water. In spite of this, the end results can vary from one another. The two samples can, however, serve as a basis. The lower acidification (recognizable by the higher pH value) when using Sucanat was by the way easy to tell by taste as well as by pH indicators, and this was so in several experiments.

In conclusion, I should like to summarize my present opinion thus:

- For household use, where other criteria matter, I can thoroughly recommend Sucanat whole cane sugar as well as honey as an alternative to white sugar, in cases where a sweetening agent cannot be dispensed with.
- I would no longer use Sucanat whole cane sugar for Kombucha, however, as here pure neutral white sugar gives a better fermentation result, and on account of its almost complete transformation into other substances is in no way injurious to health.

Note:

The suitability of other sorts of sugar (fructose etc.) is discussed in the chapter on "Can diabetics drink kombucha?"

How about using honey in the preparation of kombucha?

Honey enjoys a considerably higher reputation among health-conscious people and often replaces refined sugar as a sweetening agent.

When using honey:

1. You should be more sparing with honey when you are using it as a sweetening agent, because otherwise the strong individual taste of the honey will mask the flavor of whatever you are sweetening it with.

2. Honey is a pure natural product and in contrast to sugar contains additional vital elements.

Honey is not recommended without reservation for health cookery, however. Incidentally, according to Dr. Bruker (Der Gesundheitsberater (The Health Counselor), No. II/88), honey as well as refined sugar can render a diet of fresh fruit and vegetables and whole meal products indigestible.

The first point, that one should in general be more sparing with honey, cannot be proposed for the preparation of kombucha, because honey and sugar are not being used here as sweetening agents but for the production of the nutrient substratum, and this is prepared according to precise recommendations as to the amounts to be used, and has little to do with taste. The requirements of the microorganisms in the culture are given primary consideration, and the amounts of sugar or honey as the case may be are quantitatively geared to this.

As for the second pro-honey point, the situation is thus:

Honey contains over 100 different active and aromatic substances, and supplies the body, even if in very small amounts, with vital substances. For this reason, it has been employed as a remedy since time immemorial. Nevertheless, it consists of 70 to 80 per cent invert sugar. That is a mixture of glucose and fructose resulting from the inversion (splitting) of saccharose. This splitting of cane sugar into its individual molecules of glucose and fructose is also carried out during the fermentation process of kombucha. The sugar could not ferment otherwise.

According to Belitz and Grosch (1985) the predominant sugar in honey is fructose, averaging 38%, and glucose, averaging 31%. Other monosaccharides have as yet not been found. In addition to this, more than 20 oligosaccharides have been identified up to now. Quantitatively, maltose heads the list of the oligosaccharides.

Moreover, **opinions diverge considerably about whether honey can be used** instead of sugar when preparing kombucha. The volatile oils in the honey allegedly alter the kombucha culture considerably, at least in the long run. It must also be borne in mind that among the more than a hundred different vital and aromatic substances in honey, which are otherwise desirable, there are also substances which repress and destroy bacteria, and prevent their growth.

According to Belitz and Grosch (1985, p. 669) the bacteriostatic effect of honey can be traced to the hydrogen peroxide which is formed by the enzymatic oxidation of glucose. "Inhibine" was previously considered responsible for this.

The bacteriostatic effect certainly speaks for the wholesomeness of honey. Yet, what happens when these substances inhibit the microorganisms in the kombucha culture and prevent their vital functions? There have been people who announced with a beaming smile: "It works with honey, too." Everything went well for a while and then, after a year, the culture's activity came to a standstill.

Of course you can try to accustom the culture slowly to honey. **Microorganisms possess a high adaptability to alteration** in conditions. The great range of yeasts is mentioned by Henneberg (1926, p. 4 and 6):

"It has to be accepted that no yeast cell is absolutely like another. (...) The cause of the variations often cannot be stated; in many cases it lies e.g. in the kind of nutrition and reaction of the nutrient substratum. (...) The yeast accustoms itself gradually to the circumstances concerned. (...) Nearly all modifications brought about by special conditions during cultivation disappear rapidly as soon as the circumstances are returned to 'normal'. If the special conditions of cultivation last for a longer time, then the newly acquired characteristics are temporarily heritable. The former kind of variation can be designated as 'modification', the latter as 'fluctuation', in contrast to a third, the so-called 'mutation'. Here new, hereditary characteristics suddenly appear, seemingly for no particular reason.

Prof. Dittrich (1975) also mentions that to a certain extent it is possible for microorganisms to gain new living space for themselves, in that for example they accustom themselves in time to a new nutrient, i.e. they adapt. At the same time, with the development of new living space, sudden alterations in heredity (mutations) can occur which enable the microorganisms to achieve new things.

To what extent an adaptation or a mutation could take place and to what extent the metabolic products which pass into the beverage would then also be altered, cannot be calculated in the case of a living organism like the kombucha culture. Each person can decide for themselves whether they want to use honey or sugar. As a precaution when experimenting, however, I would always keep a reserve culture in black tea sweetened with sugar, as an insurance, so to speak, just in case the experiment should prove unsuccessful.

The proportion of the various acids in the fermented kombucha beverage would certainly be altered when honey is used. For instance, Hermann (1928) and Wiechowski (1928) demonstrated that gluconic acid (and presumably also glucuronic acid) are formed in large amounts from glucose. From fructose on the other hand, acetic acid is chiefly formed. And Danielova (1954) established that the accumulation of antibacterial substances is greater with glucose and less marked in nutrient solutions with fructose.

Now, as the proportion of fructose in honey (34-41%) predominates over the proportion of glucose (28-35%), it can be concluded that more acetic acid and less gluconic acid is formed in honey-kombucha than in sugar-kombucha. Fructose and glucose are present in equal parts in cane sugar.

At any rate, it is a fact that sugar has been used almost without exception in both past and recent experiments. Even Dr. Sklenar tried many experiments in his 30 years of experience with cultures and ultimately arrived at his recipe using black tea and normal white sugar. I think it advisable to let oneself be guided by the results of long years of research by an expert, instead of playing around experimenting with honey.

I do not want to conceal the fact that this advice conflicts with the experiences of people I know to be reliable, who claim that no recognizable difference between the use of sugar and honey has been discovered. Many people put forward the fact that a kombucha beverage of particularly aromatic character is obtained by using honey. I personally consider the taste of kombucha to be a secondary issue. The health aspect should be of primary importance. Other advocates of the use of honey state that the mucin in the honey had positive effects on the kombucha tea.

I am aware that I cannot convince many advocates of a healthy way of life with my anti-honey arguments, because the idea that "honey is good, sugar is bad" (just as "herbal tea is good, black tea is bad") is so deeply rooted in their consciousness that they cannot bring themselves to suddenly change their ways where making kombucha is concerned. And I know that many people simply want to make kombucha tea with honey from personal conviction. I'd like to meet these readers half way and at least give a couple of tips:

As far as weight is concerned, you should use rather more honey than you would sugar, because the proportion of sugar in honey, depending on the type of honey, lies between 70 and 80% only. 100 grams of honey consequently corresponds 70-80 grams cane sugar, 125 grams honey to about 90-100 grams sugar. You don't need to use expensive honey. It can be a cheap mixture of different honeys. The important thing about the quality of the honey is that it should be extracted cold and not heated above 40 °C. In contrast to sugar, the honey should only be added when the tea has cooled down to lukewarm, as otherwise the constituent substances (which you set great store by, of course) will be damaged.

Part 9
Life, cultivation, propagation, morphology

How long does the kombucha culture remain alive and active?

If the nutrients in the liquid are used up, the culture stops growing, but does not die off; it will become active once more with the addition of sugar (Schmidt, 1979).

Schmidt quotes some instructions for cultivation which say that the culture is killed through exposure to sunlight, from being scalded, and from the effects of frost. With regard to scalding, I agree unreservedly. Putting the culture into tea that is too hot can just kill it immediately. The exposure to sunlight damages the culture, which is why the fermentation container should not stand in bright sunlight but in shadow or in a dark place, is discussed above. Opinions are divided concerning the damaging effects of frost, especially as many people even deep-freeze the culture. Henneberg (1926, Vol. 1, p.6): "Cold does not generally kill off fungi. Bacteria, yeasts, mold spores can remain viable for a long time in ice. Even a temperature of -113° does not kill yeast."

Wiechowski (1928) mentions that "the growth of the kombucha symbiont and consequently a further increase in acidity" comes to an end after a more or less long time". The length of time would depend on the different circumstances under which the kombucha culture grows. He considers it "not improbable that the degree of acidity, which represents a direct gauge of the state of growth of the culture, is at the same time an indicator of a specific amount of the therapeutically active substance." Wiechowski considers the observation and recording of the increase in acidity to be the only objective means of judging the condition of the culture.

Let old mushrooms retire

Bazarewski (1915) gives the following indications for assessing the state of health of the culture: "With fresh and strong specimens of the 'Miracle Mold', the liquid was always transparent, had a noticeably sour taste and a pleasant smell reminiscent of apples. In all cases where the culture was dying off, however, there was a neutral or alkaline reaction in the liquid and an unpleasant smell as if it were going rotten, i.e. all the signs of the beginning of decomposition." To avoid confusion, I'd like to add that the above-mentioned transparency of the beverage only occurs when the fermentation container is left to stand in a quiet place for some time, and the yeast cell accumulate on the bottom. If the yeast cells are stirred up, for example when bottling the beverage, then the liquid looks a little cloudy at first. Only when the yeast cells have settled at the bottom of the bottle again does the kombucha beverage regain its clear transparent aspect.

The alkaline reaction and insufficient acidity mentioned by Wiechowski and Bazarewski can easily be checked with a pH indicator, if the taste has not already proved it. Further details about this can be found in the chapter "When is the kombucha beverage ready?"

Irion (1944) writes about the lifespan of a kombucha culture and says that if the culture is handled correctly, it can be used from four to six months and will produce 200 to 300 liters of beverage. The culture is spent and must be renewed as soon as the beverage becomes too sour, or if mold begins to form on the skin of the culture, or if brown wrinkled patches appear which tear easily. Small amounts of mold can easily be removed by dabbing the spot with ordinary table vinegar.

According to the directions of the Chemical and Bacteriological Laboratory of the Yeast Institute, Kitzingen, quoted by Arauner (1928), "you can manage for 2-3 months with a piece of culture. If the surface of the skin on the culture shows dark brown wrinkled patches which tear easily, then this is a sign that the culture is beginning to die off, is losing its effectiveness and is of no further use. The old culture must then be removed and a new culture started off."

You will probably have noticed that the over-acidity of an outworn culture mentioned by Irion seems to contradict the information given by Wiechowski and Bazarewski. And Henneberg (1926) also writes: "A disadvantage of the gradual thickening of the skin on the culture is the slow acidification and the slight sinking." He therefore recommends the timely cultivation of a new culture.

Kombucha is a life-long companion

The kombucha culture has in fact a very tough life. I've even heard of people who left the culture for months on end untended in the cellar, and then revived it by replenishing the nutrient solution. Whether it still works well or not, an older culture will in the course of time look rather unsightly. Through the effect of the tannic acid in the tea, the yeast deposit, and the dye from the various kinds of tea which has colored it, the culture grows browner and browner and can finally become as brown as café au lait.

You really mustn't let it come to the point mentioned above, viz. that your culture is beginning to die off. It's better to use fresh young cultures obtained by timely propagation. You'll find more about this in the next chapter. So you should part from an old culture in good time and without qualms. If you follow this principle, the culture can, with careful handling and clean working methods, really give you life-long joy, because like any living organism it constantly rejuvenates and propagates itself. In this way, you will always have strong cultures capable of producing vigorous fermentation. Dr. Bing (1928) emphasizes that the characteristic metabolism of the various microorganisms in the kombucha culture, "upon which the therapeutic effect is based", is bound up with the living cells of this symbiosis and can only be fully carried out by good fresh cultures capable of vigorous fermentation. Bing (1928) writes in "Die

Medizinische Welt" (The Medical World): "... cultures over three months old lose a great deal of their effectiveness, probably principally because the vitality of the culture suffers through the accumulation of its own metabolic products."

If, in spite of these constant rejuvenation measures, you should discover an abnormality in the fermentation process one day, for example, that the beverage is no longer acidifying properly, then you should think about what could have caused it. In many cases, it's a matter of unfavorable environmental influences, e.g. the effect of too much heat, exposure to sunlight, infections caused by dirty working methods, insufficient ventilation or poor quality water. Insufficient nutrition of the microorganisms is often the reason for the culture varying, mutating or degenerating. This can occur if, from a unfounded fear of using too much sugar (unfounded because the culture "eats up" all the sugar), the culture is put onto famine rations. The undernourished, exhausted, "famished" cultures resulting from this degenerate and can neither carry out their normal work of fermentation nor form sufficient new cells. If it is not already too damaged, such a culture can regenerate again as soon as it is once more given normal conditions and proper nutriment.

Begin with new cultures in good time
Henneberg (1926, Vol. 1, p. 6 ff.) explains in an article on the physiology of yeasts, that the yeast cell must absorb nourishment to build up their cell body, replenish the substances excreted through the constantly on-going metabolism, and acquire the energy needed to live. He continues: "If the yeast has too little suitable nitrogen in its nutrient solution, it breaks down its own protein reserves, which exist in abundance in well-nourished cells." The cells then appear emaciated when you look at them through the microscope, and the cell nuclei are a lot less full. According to Henneberg, after the death of the cell, even the actual cell plasma is broken down (autolysis).

Henneberg's explanations refer to yeast, However, because a considerable proportion of the kombucha culture also consists of yeast, it is surely permissible to relate these remarks, which are at least partly analogous, to the kombucha culture as well. This would also surely explain the observation that expiring cultures first cease to acidify and then finally "eat themselves up".

If you should have a kombucha culture which has degenerated through unfavorable environmental influences and which can't be regenerated again by an improvement in its living conditions, it is advisable to start again with a new culture. Otherwise, it really is always much better to use new cultures and to part from the old ones in good time. Then, the question as to how long the kombucha culture can live becomes entirely irrelevant and the apparently rather bold statement, "the kombucha culture will prove to be a lifelong companion", is true.

Cultivation and propagation of the culture

Any person, starting a career as a kombucha fan, will start small, just as many others have done before them. As basic starting material they will receive a culture and start it off to ferment in let's say two liters of tea. After 8 to 10 days their beverage is ready to drink, and they brew two more liters and put the same culture back into the fermentation container. Yet, one day, they will realize that they want to drink more than two liters of kombucha between the peaks when the beverage matures, or that other members of the family want to drink this delicious beverage, too. Now is the time to propagate the culture. There are three possible ways of doing this:

1. If the culture remains floating on the surface of the tea, it first of all grows out sideways and gradually covers the surface of the liquid completely. Then it begins to grow in depth. It can now be cut with clean scissors into small pieces about 6 cm in diameter. In doing so, care must be taken not to damage or tear the upper layer, as this would be detrimental to the growth and development of the culture.

Should the culture have grown in layers, the uppermost layer of the culture can be separated from the layers underneath (pull apart carefully) and several culture membranes of varying ages can thereby be obtained. The lowest layer is the oldest, and can be thrown away when enough new cultures have grown. In this way the culture will be constantly renewed. Mollenda (1928) recommends this procedure too: "The kombucha culture grows from above, which means that new layers are always forming on the surface, and the older layers are displaced downward. As soon as these layers turn dark brown, they must be removed, which is easily done, for if they are left stuck to the underside of the culture, the result will be a deterioration of the beverage on the one hand, and the slow death of the culture on the other."

However, these layers don't come apart as easily as Mollenda says. In many places they may have grown together completely. In this case you may need to use a sharp knife.

The formation of the layers, which are also called lamella, is due to the fact that whenever a new fermentation process is begun, the whole skin of the culture or just parts of it easily sink below the surface of the tea. A new skin then forms on top of the old one. Depending on how much space there is available on the surface of the liquid, the individual layers either remain more or less separate or else grow together in one piece. Thus several layers build up on top of one another.

2. The culture can however sink right down to the bottom of the fermentation container and remain lying there. One can't draw up any hard and fast rules as to why this should be so on some occasions, yet quite different on others. Air bubbles caught in the membrane of the culture, the quality of the water (hard/soft, surface tension) and other factors must certainly play some part in this. It also sometimes occurs that the culture first sinks down and then after a few days gets pushed up again because of the build-up of carbon dioxide bubbles which collect underneath it.

When the culture sinks to the bottom, a new culture forms on the surface of the tea. Professor Lindau's original culture (1913) sank at first to the bottom of the container. In the Report of the German Botanical Society, Prof. Lindau describes the development of a new culture thus: "When a small piece of an older culture is put into fresh nutrient solution, it sinks to the bottom (Note: not always) and remains lying there for the time being. Then, by slightly shaking the dish, mucous-like and quite irregularly formed transparent pieces can be seen spreading from the piece of culture membrane throughout the liquid. These grow bigger and reach the surface of the liquid. It takes 2-3 weeks for the development to reach this stage. From now on, the formation of the characteristic skin takes place. A colorless skin begins to emerge which looks at first as if it is sprinkled with moisture, and has a dull sheen. If the layer is lifted up, it can be seen that it is not a simple mold skin but a firm flexible covering which penetrates the liquid to a depth of 2-5 mm. Within the liquid it has the consistency of a jelly-like but very glutinous mass which cannot be ripped with a needle, but can only be cut with scissors or knife."

The culture forming on the surface consists at first of a thin skin, which gets thicker and thicker as time goes on. The speed of growth depends on various factors, such as temperature, nutrient substratum, quality of the water, and so on. Under favorable conditions, a usable new culture can have already formed by the end of the fermentation process. If the newly formed culture membrane seems to you to still be too thin after the usual fermentation period, however, you can fill a second fermentation glass with tea into which you then put only the young culture. It would be best if you put rather more sugar than usual in this "cultivation glass", so that the culture gets enough nutriment for its growth. Now leave this cultivation glass alone until the culture has reached a suitable thickness. It is important to acidify the tea in this glass, too, with at least 10% of ready prepared kombucha beverage (more would do no harm).

Should this second culture also sink to the bottom, a third culture will form on the surface of the tea, which you can then leave in peace to grow.

I'll add a couple of tips to the aforementioned method of cultivation:

If you have an older culture, it's better if a young culture forms on the surface which hasn't grown together with the older culture. The best way of achieving that is if the old culture sinks to the bottom. If it won't do you this favor, you can oblige it to do so by means of a clean pebble sterilized in scalding water.

You could also cut a nice culture into smaller pieces and let the individual bits spread out over the surface of the liquid. It's best to transfer the little pieces of culture skin into the new solution with a clean spoon that has the bowl bent at right angles to the handle. Lower the spoon with the little bits of culture skin vertically into the liquid; then draw the spoon out carefully sideways. If the pieces of culture skin sink down despite inserting them so carefully, you can prevent them from submerging by placing little slices of thoroughly boiled cork under them. Thin slices can be cut from a wine-bottle cork e.g. with an electric bread-slicer.

In Henneberg (1926, Vol. 1, p. 537) I found another tip, that the formation of a skin may be hastened by "using a glass rod to crush a few bits of skin around the sides of the container at the surface level of the solution." This tip in fact applies to wine-vinegar bacteria, but could also be useful for kombucha cultivation.

3. With the third method of propagation, you can make use of the fact that **ready-fermented kombucha is biologically active** (provided that the beverage is not sterilized, which you're not going to do for domestic use). There are namely still a great many living micro-organisms in the beverage which are capable of further development.

For this method, you pour part of the ready-fermented kombucha beverage into a clean glass and cover it lightly. Then let it stand at a temperature as near the optimum as possible. In the course of a few days a thin skin forms on the surface of the liquid, which as with the other methods, gets thicker and thicker and is soon firm enough to be carefully transferred to a new infusion of sweetened tea. This method takes a bit longer than the other two for a new culture to form.

After a while, you may also discover a new, small culture floating on the surface of the liquid in the bottles you've filled, which has developed despite the lack of oxygen. This is evidence of the great biological activity of kombucha and its ability to survive in the most adverse circumstances.

You can add the young self-propagated cultures to the parent culture in the same glass. You can consequently put several cultures into one fermentation container, gradually increase the size of the containers, or else use several fermentation containers.

The culture, as a living organism, is dependent on outward conditions for its development. Because of this, it doesn't always react in the same way – just as no apple looks exactly like another. The culture can sometimes look more transparent and jelly-like, at other times more whitish, gray, brownish or peach-colored. This depends among other things on whether the yeasts or the bacterial components are working the most. Its color naturally very much depends on what sort of tea is being used.

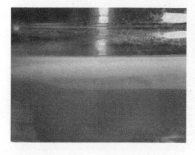

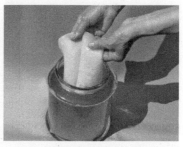

If the culture floats on the surface of the liquid, it gradually covers the surface completely. It gets the form of the surface of the glass

Should the culture have grown in layers, the uppermost layer can be separated from the layers underneath (pull apart carefully)

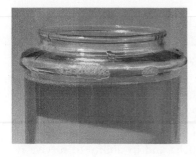

When the culture sinks to the bottom, a new culture forms on the surface of the tea.

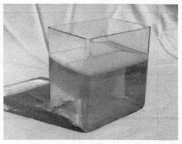

The kombucha beverage is biologically active. Pour part of ready-fermented beverage into a glass. In the course of a few days a new skin forms on the surface of the liquid.

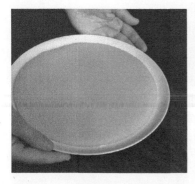

This new kombucha culture has been grown in a round glass. You can cut the large layer into smaller pieces with scissors and transfer the little pieces into more fermentation containers. Thus, you may increase the production of the beverage.

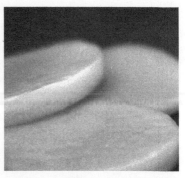

If you have got enough kombucha babies, pass them on to your friends. Always include ready -fermented beverage (the starter liquid) and complete information, preferably this book.

Does a large quantity of culture influence fermentation results and growth?

When a great many new cultures have been raised, and their vigorous growth threatens to swamp you, the question will one day arise: is there any advantage in putting as many cultures as possible into the fermentation container?

The question of the influence of the "seed quantity" also preoccupied Professor Henneberg (1926 Volume 1, p. 239). In his experiments with yeast, he established that with 0.8 to 2% seed, all the cells sprouted. The more he increased the amount of seed, the fewer cells sprouted. With 12% seed, none of the cells sprouted at all. The size of the daughter cells were also smaller, the denser the seed. So a large quantity of seed increasingly stunts the sprouting process. Schön (1978, p.50) confirms that the growth rate is reduced through a high density of the corresponding microorganisms.

The conclusions drawn by Sakaryan and Danielova (1948) tend to be along the same lines. They conducted the following experiment to elicit the dependence of the infusion activity on the volume of the nutrient solution: five glass containers of equal size were taken and filled with 100, 250, 500, 750 and 1000 ml of nutrient solution. A piece of culture of equal size and weight was placed in each glass. Irrespective of the different quantities of liquid, on the fifth day of growth the pH value was the same in all containers (2.8). The pH value did not change, then. The effectiveness (the activity against disease bacteria) continued to increase, however. On the 8th day, the sample with 100 ml of nutrient solution proved to be the most actively effective, whereas the four other samples, despite the varying amounts of liquid, were about equally actively effective. The Russian scientists conclude from this that the activity of the infusion is almost independent of the volume of the nutrient solution. It is indeed possible that the effectiveness of the infusion in the first few days of growth varies in strength according to the varying amounts of liquid, but this is evened out over a longer period of cultivation (8-18 days).

The experiments of the two Russian scientists also proved that the activity of the infusion is not only dependent on the formation of acids, but also on other substances, the amounts of which gradually increase over a longer period of cultivation.

Despite the pH value remaining the same (on the 5th, 8th and 18th day), the effectiveness of the kombucha beverage is of varying strength. The activity of the solution does, in fact, decrease after the neutralization of the beverage by means of various alkaline solutions, but does not disappear. Even high temperatures (50 and 100 °C) have, according to these tests, "no influence whatever on the activity of the kombucha infusion." (This insensitivity to high temperatures naturally relates only to the antibacterial properties of the fermented beverage, not to the yeast cells etc. suspended in the beverage, and not to the culture itself.)

As there seems to be no advantage therefore in putting vast amounts of culture into one fermentation container, it is advisable to part from older cultures in good time and always to use one of the youngest. That doesn't mean to say that only one culture per glass should be used, but there's no added advantage in overdoing it.

What happens during the process of propagation?

The kombucha culture consists of various yeasts and bacteria which live together to their mutual benefit and form a sort of symbiosis. In contrast to the genus of the basidiomycetes, such as boletus, mushroom, chanterelle etc., bacteria (previously called schizomycetes) and yeasts (ascomycetes) do not propagate themselves by means of spores, but have another form of reproduction, which I will now explain briefly.

Bacteria

In single-cells microorganisms the simplest form or reproduction is by division (fission). Bacteria, which reproduce by this method, were therefore previously classified as fission fungi. Under the present classification system, bacteria are placed in a class of their own as prokaryotes (without a typical nucleus), as distinct from plants and animals. Around 1600 kinds of bacteria are known. The reproduction of bacteria is always carried out asexually by means of binary fission. The period between one fission and another is mostly only 15 to 40 minutes (according to Ahlheim, 1967).

The fission is initiated by the appearance of a wall across the middle. In elongated types, it always runs at right angles to the longitudinal axis and splits later on (Garms, 1964). Bacteria require warmth, food and water. Some require oxygen (aerobic bacteria), others live wholly or partly without oxygen (anaerobic bacteria).

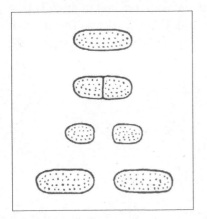

Reproduction of bacteria by binary fission

Yeasts (Saccharomyces)

The generic term for yeast plants is saccharomyces, which includes the important species of culture yeasts with a pronounced fermentative ability. The name comes from the Greek word mucus, which means fungus. The first part of the word comes from the Greek sakharon (= sugar). So the word saccharomyces could be translated as "sugar-eating fungus". The yeasts are also classified as belonging to the ascomycetes. We won't go into further details of their position within the system here. What can be of importance to us towards understanding the connection with the preparation and cultivation of kombucha, is the type of reproduction. Whereas, most of the yeasts reproduce vegetatively by means of budding. Baker's yeast, distiller's yeast, and brewer's yeast are like this. In addition, there is the combination of budding and fission (saccharomycodes). The fission yeasts, which we will go into below, reproduce by means of fission. Only in rare cases can sporulation also be observed in yeasts.

All the types of yeast that have been found in the kombucha culture, with the exception of Schizosaccharomyces pombe, reproduce by means of budding. The cells bulge out like a ball in one place, the nucleus divides, and a daughter cell segments itself off. With a good supply of food and oxygen, the yeast will bud in several places simultaneously. The daughter cells on their part bud again, and real little cell colonies come into being (Garms, 1964). The budding may be bipolar at both ends or multipolar in all directions (Schmidt, 1979).

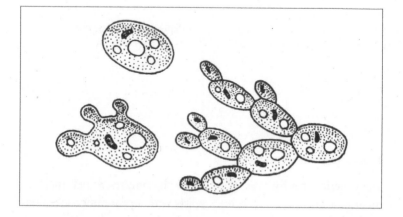

Reproduction of yeasts by budding. Young cells segmenting themselves off.

Fission yeasts (Schizosaccharomyces)

There is a small group of yeasts, the fission yeasts, which reproduce by means of binary fission. The cells don't bud as with most of the other yeasts, but divide in a similar manner to bacteria into two independent new organisms. The pombe fission yeast (Schizosaccharomyces pombe), which is also contained in the kombucha culture, belongs to this type. According to Schmidt)1979) the cells are cylindrical and form a wall across the middle at the time of fission. Scars remain after the fission by which they can be additionally recognized.

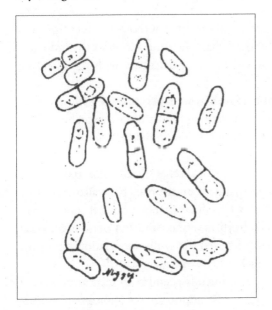

Pombe fission yeast (Schizosaccharomyces pombe). The cells do not bud but divide like bacteria. Cells from the fermentation of spices. Simple preparation (1000 x).

(Ref. HENNEBERG, Handbuch der Gärungsbakteriologie, Vol. 2, 1926, publ. by Paul Parey, Berlin & Hamburg.)

The "genuine" kombucha culture

"Have I got the real kombucha culture? Where do I get the right culture from?" These are questions that bother a lot of people, and are forever cropping up.

To come straight to the point: there is not one clear answer to this question. Reiss (1987) reduces it to the common denominator: "The precise combination of the component elements of individual kombucha preparations can vary widely, so that it's not so much a case of 'the' kombucha culture, but of a great number of them."

This view is confirmed by all the other authors. Lindner (1913 and 1917/18) had already noticed that the composition of the individual cultures could be very different, particularly with regard to the yeasts.

In addition, Valentin (1930), who experimented with a variety of different strains, says the varying results of his researches taught him that there is a great variety in the individual culture colonies. He describes his results in the following terms:

"At any rate, it must be emphasized that the chemical processes in kombucha cultures are dependent on the bacteria available. But it's not just from the fermented products that one can tell commercially obtainable kombucha cultures contain a variety of quite different strains of yeast and bacteria; even the symbiotic relationship of the individual varieties to each other varies greatly."

Valentin (1928) even recommends chemists to raise a varieties of cultures, to be able to give their customers the appropriate culture to match the desired taste.

The Russian research scientist Danielova confirms in a thesis published in 1954 (Morphology of the tea fungus) that the actual composition of the symbiont varies according to geographical and climatic conditions, and depends on whatever types of wild yeasts and bacteria exist locally.

The variety of combinations forming the kombucha culture can possibly be caused by differing growth of the individual constituents.

Depending on which conditions of growth best suit which constituents of the culture, so one sort develops better than another.

As I considered the question of the "genuine" kombucha culture to be very important, I consulted Professor Ulf Stahl of the Technical University, Berlin (Microbiological Research Institute), who was known to me as an authority in the field of microbiology. Professor Stahl told me that the opinion of the Microbiological Research Institute is that the kombucha culture is composed of Schizosaccharomyces pombe and Acetobacter xylinum.

These constituents are also given by authors worldwide. Dr. Maxim Bing (1928) gives Bacterium xylinum and the tropical Pombe yeast, as well as Bact. xylonoides and gluconicum as constituents in pure cultures. The first two are given a certain prominence.

Dr. Arauner (1929) confirms this: "The kombucha culture is not a standardized thing, but a fungal consortium of Bacterium xylinum (former designation of Acetobacter xylinum) in symbiosis with Pombe yeast."

Prof. Henneberg (1926 b) also mentions exactly the same combination in his handbook on fermentation bacteriology, and recommends pure cultures of both these constituents.

A pure or axenic culture consists of a single type of microorganism. In bacteriology, often only the descendants of one single bacterium cell (isolation of single-cell colonies) are referred to as a pure culture (Schön, 1978).

When Prof. Henneberg recommends using pure cultures, he means by that nothing more than cultivating both constituent part – Bacterium xylinum and the Pombe yeast – separately, and only then bringing them together. Preparing the beverage at home, of course, one has to continue working with the already combined constituents of the culture.

To sum up, one may say: The principal constituents Schizosaccharomyces pombe and Bacterium (Acetobacter) xylinum are both confirmed beyond doubt in the writings of the experts. An exception to this is Wiechowski (1928), who considers Bacterium gluconicum to be the principal bacterium and Bacterium xylinum second in order of importance. Irrespective of these, other bacteria and yeasts are mentioned as being constituent elements, whose presence however varies.

Our opinions are like our watches.
Nobody's is exactly the same as
anybody else's, and yet everyone
believes their own to be right.
Christian Fürchtegott Gellert

The origin of the kombucha culture

Nobody knows exactly how the first kombucha culture came into being. There are some guesses and ideas about how the kombucha originated – namely the symbiosis of bacteria and yeasts. The mushroom was propagated in the past by pieces of skin, which were planted in nutritional solutions and then passed on from hand to hand. There was no evidence of a new spontaneous generation.

Many yeasts exist on fruits and elsewhere, it is therefore easy to imagine that through the action of air currents or insects that the bacteria of the mushroom and the yeasts were brought together so that they could develop together. Such an assumption that these events occurred by chance was also had by Lindner (1913, 1917/1918).

Certain microorganisms that exist in the kombucha also exist in the sap of bleeding trees. This is how spontaneous developments of kombucha in teas that are left standing could be possible as insects could carry them from the neighborhood wounds of trees or flowers as agents of fermentation and bacteria that produce acids.

Dinslage and Ludorff wrote in 1927:

"Even if the Bacterium Xylinum (a component of the culture of kombucha, nowadays called Acetobacter Xylinum) is frequent fungus on bleeding oaks and the transmission of it through fruit flies (Drosophila melanogaster) to a tea with sugar is plausible, it would be very unlikely that the necessary yeast would also be present. A much simpler explanation would be one similar to that of kefir which was produced by accident through a fungal symbiosis and then continued to spread."

A little about the history of kombucha

Kombucha is nothing new. Lightly fermented tea is an ancient home-made folk remedy. For generations its efficacy has been held in high regard by many nations, especially those of eastern Asia. The original source of this symbiosis of bacteria and yeasts is said to have come from China or Japan. It is reported that the culture was discovered in the Chinese Empire more than 2000 years ago.

The use of the kombucha tea mushroom, thought to have originated in the Far East, penetrated some time ago into Russia. At the time of the First World War, use of the kombucha mushroom spread further westward. Russian and German POWs seem to have played a significant role in its dissemination. By the mid-twenties, this tea mushroom was already widespread in Germany as a home and folk remedy. Dr. Harms (1927) remarked that, in some parts of Germany, for example in the Westphalian industrial region, the tea mushroom was already widely used. "The mushroom is eagerly sought after in certain circles, and is gladly passed on to others." In the inter-war years, the tea mushroom found wide distribution in Germany, and was sold in pharmacies under a number of fanciful names such as "Mo-Gu" or "Fungojapon."

All knowledge of the kombucha culture was forgotten about for a long time. This was due to the uncertainties of World War II, when there was a scarcity of tea and sugar, the raw materials needed to make it. The present trend towards a return to natural foodstuffs, remedies and luxuries has re-awakened widespread interest in the valuable natural remedy kombucha and its preparation and cultivation. Many naturopaths and general practitioners recommend kombucha to their patients as a natural healing treatment.

What other names have been given to the kombucha culture?

Because of its widespread use, each folk group has given this popular beverage a name of their own. Thus, the culture bears many other names in addition to "Kombucha".

What is certain is that the word "**kombucha**", which comes from the Japanese, has actually been erroneously used to designate the culture. "Kombu" is the name of a brown seaweed (Laminaria japonica, probably also other types), which is used in Japan as a foodstuff (Tschirch, 1912, from Steiger and Steinegger, 1957) or else as tea. "Cha" means tea. "Kombucha" is therefore tea obtained from this seaweed (Steiger and Steinegger, 1957). Probably the tea was made with seaweed tea, and the name of the tea was transferred to the fermented tea beverage obtained from it and finally to the culture itself (Meixner, 1983).

The beverage got the name "**tea kvass**" from kvass, which is also a rather sharp, sparkling, refreshing beverage that has come to us from the east by way of Russia, but which has nothing to do with kombucha. The popular Russian drink kvass is produced by lactic acid fermentation of bread soaked in water, to which various other ingredients have been added according to whatever recipe is being used, such as malt, flour, syrup, sugar peppermint. etc.

From the following list of further names that have been given to the culture, a great deal can be learned about its origins and also about how it has helped people. It can be immediately seen from many of the names, that the origin of the culture presumably lies in the east: China, Japan, Manchuria, Russia, India. The description "**jellyfish**" or "**medusa**" is scientifically untenable. The culture has nothing to do with that. The description "**Champignon de longue vie**" (= long life mushroom) is also used outside France and indicates the healing power and possibility of lengthening life attributed to the culture.

The name "**Heldenpilz**" (hero's mushroom) comes from the fact that the culture used to be handed out to Japanese warriors. They kept the culture in their field flasks, and by continually adding freshly brewed tea to it, they made themselves a beverage that was refreshing and at the same time strengthening because of its vitamin content (Popiel, 1917).

The culture was called "**Olinka**" in Bohemian and Moravian monasteries. Hermann (1929) writes that it was allegedly cultivated in the monasteries long before it was even known in the surrounding areas. It was a strictly guarded secret, and the culture was given the name "Olinka", probably as a cover-up. By asking "How is Olinka faring?" one could secretly enquire after the prosperity of the culture. Then it was apparently brought out of the monasteries and found its way into a few noble families (Hermann, 1929). Steiger and Steinegger (1957) point out that it seems the learned monasteries formerly often knew and practiced many more things than were known about by the local peasants, citizens, and even nobility. Such things were kept strictly to oneself. One has only to think of the art of brewing beer, the production of liqueur, the baking of ergot-free bread – bread which would no longer make people ill – etc.

The name "**Kombucha**" occurs particularly in articles from Czechoslovakia, for instance in Moravian Ostrau (Pletnitzky, 1927) and Haida in Bohemia (Meissner, 1928) in answer to questions in periodicals. "**Fungus japonicus**" is given here as the botanical name. At the end of the 20's, a few chemists put the culture on the market under imaginary names like "**Mo-Gû**" or "**Fungojapon**" (Steiger and Steinegger, 1957).

In the 20-volume Brockhaus Encyclopedia (17th edition, 1970, Wiesbaden), the kombucha culture is quoted in the tenth volume under the heading "**Kombucha, Japanese tea-sponge, tea fungus.**"

In 1973 the name "**Combucha**" was accorded an entry in the 4th new edition of Hager's Handbook of Pharmaceutical Practice for chemists, drug manufacturers, doctors, and medical officers of health (Volume IV, pp. 254-256). This is an 8-volume basic reference work on pharmaceutical practice, which can be consulted at any chemist's. The name kombucha or Combucha is in general mainly used today.

The name "**Kargasok tea**" apparently originates from the following event: "About 60 years ago a Japanese woman discovered many people in Kargasok (Russia) who were over 100 years old. Old and young alike drank tea fermented with the kombucha culture every day. The Japanese woman took the preparation, which was said to confer immortality on the drinker, back home with her. Dr. Pan Pen later wrote a report on the experiments he had been conducting for years: Kargasok tea definitely prolongs life, cures chicken-pox and shingles, reduces wrinkles, prevents cancer, averts menopause, improves vision, strengthens the leg muscles, cures sweaty feet, constipation, diarrhea, joint and back pains, ulcers, hardening of the arteries, diabetes, cataract, heart attack, strengthens the kidneys, reduces gall-stones and obesity, promotes sleep, helps travel sickness and hemorrhoids, gray hair grows in dark again and bald patches grow over."

I found this story in a leaflet giving instructions on how to prepare the tea, without reference to author or source. This report seems to me to be rather strongly exaggerated. I could find no reference to a Dr. Pan Pen in any bibliography.

Synonymous names for the culture
- Brinum-Ssene (Latvian = miracle fungus)
- Cainii grib (Russian)
- Cainogo griba (Georgian)
- Cembuya orientalis (Latin)
- Chamboucho (Romanian)
- Champignon de la charité (French)
- Champignon de longue vie (French)
- Champignon japonais or chinois (French)
- Champignon miracle (French)
- Chinesischer Teepilz (German)
- Ciuperca de ceai (Romanian = tea fungus)
- Comboucha (French)

- Combucha (Japanese)
- Fungojapon (former trade name)
- Fungus japonicus (pharmaceutical name)
- Funko cinese (Italian)
- Ganoderma japonicus (literally = Japanese mushroom)
- Gichtqualle (German)
- Haipao
- Heldenpilz (German)
- Hongo (Spanish)
- Indischer Teepilz (German)
- Indischer Teeschwamm (German)
- Indischer Weinpilz (German)
- Indisch-japanischer Teepilz (German)
- Japan gomba (Hungarian)
- Japanischer Combucha (German)
- Japanischer Pilz (German)
- Japanischer Schwamm (German)
- Japanischer Teepilz (German)
- Japanisches Mütterchen (German)
- Japanpilz (German)
- Japanska gliva (Yugoslavian)
- Japonski grib (Russian = Japanese mushroom)
- Kambuha (Russian)
- Kargasok Schwamm (German)
- Kargasok-Teepilz (German)
- Kocha Kinoko (Japanese, Kocha = Black Tea, Kinoko = Mushroom or fungus
- Kinokocha (Japanese, Kinoko = Mushroom or fungus, Cha = tea)
- Kombucha (Germanized form of Japanese name, used internationally)
- Kombuchaschwamm (German)
- Kongo
- Kwassan (trade name for a former extract of the culture)
- Mandschurischer Pilz (German)

- Mandschurischer Schwamm (German)
- Mandschurisch-japanischer Pilz (German)
- Medusomyces Gisevii LINDAU (scientific name)
- Ma-Gu
- Mo-Gû (former trade name)
- Olinka (in Bohemian and Moravian monasteries)
- Red tea fungus (the Japanese use the word "red tea" for black tea)
- Russische Blume (German)
- Russische Qualle (German)
- Russischer Pilz (German)
- Sakvasska (Russian = acid)
- Symbiont schizosaccharomyces pombe – bacterium xylinum
-   (Dr. Bing, 1929, gives this name as a scientific description)
- Tea fungus Kombucha
- Tea mould (Java)
- Teekwasspilz (German)
- Teepilz (German)
- Teyi saki (Armenian)
- Teeschwamm (German)
- Thee-Schimmel (Dutch)
- Theezwam Komboecha (Dutch)
- Tschambucco
- Wolgameduse (German)
- Wolgapilz (German)
- Wolgaqualle (German)
- Wunderpilz (German)
- Yaponge
- Zauberpilz (German)

Synonymous names for the kombucha beverage
- Cainii kvass (Russian)
- Combuchagetränk (German)
- Elixir de longue vie (French)
- Komboecha-drank (Dutch)
- Kombucha-thee (Dutch)

- (In the Netherlands the name kombucha is mainly used today instead of Komboecha)
- Kombuchagetränk (German)
- Kombuchakvass (German)
- Kargasoktee (German)
- Medusentee (German)
- Russischer Tee-Essig (German)
- Tea beer
- Tea cider
- Tea wine
- Teekvass (German)
- Teemost (German)
- Theebier (Dutch)

In Chinese / Ling Tsche	In Arabian
Divine Mushroom A Chinese Professor wrote this for a friend of mine. He told me this name is used for kombucha in **China** 靈芝	(to read from right to left): *"Kombucha – the spring of wellbeing"* كمبيشا منبع الصحة والإستجمام

In Japanese	In Japanese	In Russian
紅茶キノコ **Kōcha-kinoko** With the Kombucha beverage prepared of **black tea** Kocha = black tea Kinoko = mushroom	**Kinoko-cha** With the Kombucha beverage prepared of **green tea** Kinoko = mushroom cha = tea, mushroom tea	чайный гриб chaynij grib = tea mushroom **Гриб** The kombucha beverage is called mushroom or also simply **квас** *(kvass)* although it is completely different to Brottrunk.

Part 10
Problems arising during the preparation of kombucha

Inhibition of the development of microorganisms

If you follow the instructions exactly and handle the kombucha culture with thought and care, you should hardly have any difficulties to reckon with. You don't even need to worry about harmful bacteria developing, because the acidity of the fermenting solution will prevent that.

The fact that one microorganism can inhibit the development of another is already well known. Several such protective mechanisms with which the culture fights off competitors are also to be found in kombucha.

In the realm of living things, several groups of organisms often compete for one nutrient substratum. Other microorganisms are omnipresent in kombucha too. They are in the air all around us, in the water, in the ground. Airborne spores are deposited with the dust which covers everything in a more or less thick layer. Whenever we take hold of anything, spores get onto our hands too.

Naturally, airborne spores also settle on foodstuffs and on the surface of the kombucha culture. If they find optimum living conditions there, then the food goes rotten. Mold spores are often found on food. In many cases this is Aspergillus repens. The mound forms a light green patch like a lawn closely covering the surface of the food (Dittrich, 1975, p.63). However, food is usually conserved by keeping it dry, salted, pickled, or preserved in some other way. Such means can prevent food from going bad through the development of microorganisms (Dittrich, p.35).

The preservative effect of organic acids

Acidification has been recognized from time immemorial as a means of preserving foodstuffs. There is still a place for this today, and there always will be in the future. Dr. Erich Lück (1988) writes in the Deutsche Apotheker Zeitung (German Pharmaceutical Times): "Acids have a preserving effect in that they produce a pH value in the foodstuff to be preserved, which certain microorganisms can no longer tolerate, in particular those which create toxins. However, other bacteria and most of the yeasts and molds cannot be inhibited by an acid pH value unless something else happens as well." Toxins are poisonous metabolic products.

To a certain extent, the kombucha beverage preserves itself. It produces substances, for instance, which are even listed in the 1963 EEC regulations for preservatives: acetic acid (E 260) and lactic acid (E 270). Any alien organisms are repressed through the acids it produces.

Bazarewski (1915) determined this. He examined the solution in which the kombucha culture grows and observed that the microflora was not abundant. The production of acetic acid prevents the development of any microorganisms which do not belong to the kombucha culture organism.

A similar process of self-preservation can be found in mild which is turning sour. The resulting lactic acid represses decay bacteria which would otherwise break down the protein. Similar preservative effects are found in pickled gherkins, sauerkraut, and silage. The acetic acid in pickled gherkins acts as a bactericide.

Oxalic acid is a metabolic product of many fungi, and also of many higher plants. This acid was also detected in kombucha, e.g. by Valentin (1930). The preservative effect of oxalic acid can be put to good use, for example, when bottling rhubarb. The sticks of rhubarb are simply washed and packed as tightly as possible into a preserving jar, covered with water, and hermetically sealed. They are then often still usable for cooking purposes a year later (Dittrich, 1975, p.74). Even unripe fruit, such as apples and gooseberries, don't go bad under water. The high amount of various organic acids contained in them makes them resistant to attack by bacteria (Dittrich, p.74).

The preservative effect of alcohol

The preservative effect of alcohol is universally known. Every housewife who preserves soft fruit in alcohol for Christmas knows that she must take care to keep the concentration of alcohol sufficiently high by adding high-proof rum or brandy, otherwise the fruit will begin to ferment. Food chemistry works on the basis that alcohol over 18% has a preservative effect.

Possibly less well known is the fact that even the smallest amounts of alcohol have a noticeably inhibiting effect on the growth of mold. This occurs for instance with grape must. When the grapes are pressed, all sorts of spores sticking to the fruit get into the must. They all flourish unhindered at first. But then the yeasts very quickly begin to ferment and produce alcohol. The small amount of alcohol at this initial stage is already enough to suppress the molds.

Naturally – and this is astonishing, although frequently encountered – the yeast cells inhibit their own development through their own metabolic product, viz. alcohol. However, only an alcohol content of over 15% stops the yeast from growing, and the yeast will only be killed when the alcohol in the solution rises to an even higher percentage (Dittrich, 1975).

Less astonishing than the yeasts preventing their own growth through their own metabolic products, is that the alcohol produced by the yeast works on alien bacteria and suppresses molds. Thus, the addition of a small amount of alcohol to the kombucha fermentation solution, mentioned by a few authors, apart from the intended principal purpose of supplying the acetic bacteria with nutrition right from the beginning, may also at the same time suppress the development of molds. However, the yeasts in the kombucha culture exercise their preservative function even without the additional alcohol, in that the polysaccharides, after having split into monosaccharides, are converted into alcohol and carbon dioxide.

Self-preservation of kombucha culture by means of antibiotics

The Russian Professor G. F. Barbancik (1958) in his book on the cainii grib (Russian name for the kombucha culture) attributes the success of treatments using the kombucha infusion in all cases of illness principally to its active antibiotic effect. He was also able to observe the great activity of the acetic acid bacteria (Acetobacter xylinum) in laboratory tests, when Streptococci, Diplococci, Flexner and Shigella rods were sown in the tea. This led him to the view that the acetic acid bacteria energetically suppress any other microbes surrounding them (vigorous bacterial antagonism). That is why Prof. G. Sakaryan and L. Danielova saw in this phenomenon a bactericide, and called the antibiotic excreted by the acetic acid bacteria "Bacteriocidin":

Sakaryan and Danielova (1948) mention in an article that because of the antibiotic properties of the kombucha beverage, "sterile precautionary measures" are not necessary when cultivating the culture. They continue: "The culture grows without being covered, and atmospheric air has free access. Throughout all this, the nutrient solution on which the culture grows and to which the microorganisms in the air have free access, remains transparent and unpolluted."

And I. N. Konovalov (1959), who also comes from Russia, mentions that the intensive reproduction of the kombucha yeasts and of the Bacterium xylinum noticeably suppress the proliferation of other kinds of yeast and bacteria in every culture medium.

Inhibitory effect of carbon dioxide

As already mentioned, the yeasts in the kombucha culture produce carbon dioxide as well as alcohol; it is then converted into carbonic acid under the influence of moisture. Both of these products have the effect of inhibiting the growth of alien organisms, whereas yeast tolerates considerable amounts of carbonic acid without losing its vigor.

Carbon dioxide is a gas with antimicrobial properties and is listen in the EEC regulations for preservatives as E 290. The reason for the effectiveness of gases is that they are harmful to the cells of microbes. An early reference to this means of preserving food, by the way, is to be found in the Bible (Genesis 41:35). According to this, Pharaoh ordered Joseph to store up a fifth of the grain harvest in storehouses during the seven years of plenty, to have a reserve supply for the seven years of famine. Because of the carbon dioxide resulting from respiration, the grain was protected from rotting (Lück, 1988).

In spite of the above-mentioned capacities for self-preservation found in the kombucha beverage, problems which seem genuine – and even genuine ones too – do sometimes occur, and this is explained as follows.

Problems which seem genuine but aren't

On the underside of a culture lying on the bottom of the glass, you sometimes get brownish "streamers" (as Lindau calls them) or "rat's tails" (Meixner, 1983) which hang down in the liquid of the culture is floating on the top and, as Lindau says, "lend the culture a distant similarity to a floating jelly-fish." These streamers are caused by dead and torn skins, viz. dead cells, which sometimes break loose and remain suspended in the liquid. These streamers can be washed off without difficulty under running water, and are not an indication of damage to the culture. If such streamers should get into the beverage while it is being bottled, they can easily be caught in a sieve when you pour the beverage into a glass to drink.

Slimy brownish pieces can also build up on the culture. They consist mostly of dead cells. They can be washed off with cold or lukewarm water, or carefully scraped off with a teaspoon.

If the beverage is not filtered when it is ready, it looks rather cloudy. That comes from the little pieces in suspension and the yeast which is to be found in it. There's no need to see that as a problem. Bigger bits as well as jelly-like veils or "intricate masses of mold threads" (as Lakowitz puts it, 1928), which can form even after the bottles have been filled, are also easily removed by straining through a sieve.

In particular, if the culture develops more of a whitish coloring, sometimes beginning with little islands on the surface of the liquid, then many people think it is mold. Little bubbles of carbonic acid, produced as a result of fermentation, also often form under the newly growing skin of the culture floating on the surface of the liquid. At a cursory glance these white, often foamy-looking bubbles can easily be taken for mold. These whitish patches, however, are easily recognized under a magnifying glass as "air bubbles" under the skin of the culture.

Carbonic acid bubbles can also form under older cultures floating on the surface, and they can cause the culture to bulge upwards here and there, which gives it a scarred appearance.

Genuine problems

We have heard how the kombucha culture defends itself against alien microorganisms and that these therefore hardly stand a chance of holding their own in the acid environment of the fermentation liquid. The pH value of a solution has a crucial influence on the growth of microorganisms. The regulation of a particularly suitable pH value is therefore of great importance, and this is achieved from the start of the kombucha fermentation process by a corresponding acidification.

Low pH values, like those produced by the kombucha culture, lie just outside the optimum range for molds. Sufficient acidification is therefore also an important factor in avoiding the formation of mold (which seldom happens).

Bing (1928, Die medizinische Welt) mentions that the acids formed by the kombucha culture have a strongly inhibitory (antagonistic) effect on putrefactive bacteria and mold spores. He writes: "If these are introduced into the culture, they rapidly die. It's very instructive to see what happens when mold spores are introduced into the culture in such a way that they run down from the rim of the container. They then grow into flourishing colonies above the level of the nutrient solution, but end with a clear-cut line at the point of contact with the meniscus." (According to Bing, the antagonism to putrefactive bacteria also helps in the prevention of dysentery).

What to do when mold forms

The various kinds of Aspergillus and Penicillin spores are the most widespread forms of mold. They live on a variety of substrate, e.g. on foodstuffs like bread, fruit, milk – and can also develop on a kombucha culture which has been kept under unfavorable environmental conditions, if it is inadequately protected from open sources of mold, or from spores which are present in the atmosphere. This can occur with any foodstuff. Nobody would dream of stopping eating bread on account of this, or of not making jam any more, or of banishing any other uncovered foodstuffs from their home. However, the danger of infection through alien microorganisms is greater with leftovers and uncovered drinks and foodstuffs, for instance, than with the kombucha culture, where, as has already been explained, various self-protective mechanisms function which other foodstuffs do not possess.

In spite of this, mold may grow on the kombucha culture (though this is extremely rare) just as it may grow on any foodstuff. According to Henneberg, mold forms particularly where there is an open source of mold somewhere in the room, or where spores can somehow alight on the culture. The worse the conditions provided for the yeasts and bacteria in the kombucha culture, the greater the chances of mold developing. Apparently mold is also particularly likely to form where people smoke in the same room.

If mold should nevertheless occur, it should be treated in the same way as mold on any other foodstuff. Prof. Henneberg (1926 b, p. 379) mentions in connection with the preparation of kombucha:

"Now and then the appearance of green colonies and an unpleasant smell drew one's attention to the fact that mold was forming (mostly Citromyces). Washing the skin of the culture carefully under running water and increasing the acidity with boiled vinegar proved effective here. Occasionally there were also problems with alien acetic bacteria, e.g. Bact. ascendens. In this case, a premature clouding became noticeable, and a dusty, delicate vinegar skin which crept up the sides of the container above the jelly-like culture. At the same time, there was an alteration in the aroma (formation of aldehyde), and the formation of vinegar became too strongly marked. This infection should be treated in the same way as for mold formation. The occasional appearance of film-forming yeasts (dry, whitish, powdery skin) can be removed in the same way."

The establishment of film-forming yeasts becomes noticeable when the acid, instead of increasing, decreases from day to day. This is because film-forming yeasts have a preference for feeding on acids. Film-forming yeasts with the ability to produce acids are very rare (see Henneberg, Handbuch der Gärungsbakteriologie, Vol. 1, p. 533, 1926).

Hans Irion (1944), in his "Lehrgang für Drogistenfachschulen" (p. 405), gives the following instructions regarding cases of mold forming on the kombucha culture: "Small amounts of mold may be easily removed by dabbing the area with ordinary table vinegar."

If mold should form, I consider it best to be on the safe side and start again with a new culture.

Tiresome pests: vinegar flies

Tiny vinegar flies can be particularly tiresome when you are making kombucha. They can be found, especially in the summer months when the weather is hot, on liquids containing sugar, alcohol or vinegar, or even on fruit, and they are attracted by the aromatic smell of the kombucha beverage. Their sense of smell is extraordinarily well developed. They appear suddenly, as if from nowhere, buzz around the fermentation container, settle on the cloth covering it, and try to get inside. Once they do manage to get inside, "little worms" soon begin to crawl around on the surface of the culture. These are the vinegar fly maggots which have hatched out of the eggs laid by the vinegar flies. They make the culture look very unappetizing.

Apparently Prof. Henneberg was also bothered by these little pests. He writes in detail about the "little vinegar flies", which are also known scientifically as "Drosophila fenestrarum Fallén". With kind permission of the publisher, I borrowed Professor Henneberg's descriptions, in the form of extracts from Henneberg, Handbuch der Gärungsbakteriologie, 2. Band, 1926, published by Paul Parey, Berlin and Hamburg.

On pp. 355-357, Henneberg writes among other things: "In every business and laboratory handling sweet fruit or liquids containing alcohol or vinegar, there are flies which are about ½ – ⅓ the size of a common house-fly, with a yellowish-brown colored body and vermilion eyes. These insects, described as 'vinegar flies', are to be seen, without exception, in every vinegar factory, distillery, yeast factory, fruit juice factory and so on, especially during the summer months when the weather is hot. (...) The flies are 2½ – 3 mm long. Though they may measure only half the normal size if the larvae have been undernourished. (...) The white-colored larvae (maggots) are 5 mm long and 1 mm across. On the front end of the body, which consists of twelve segments, are two black mouth-hooks. One of the principal sources of food for the maggots and flies are the areas of fungal growth formed by sheets of mold, film-forming yeasts or acetic bacteria on the surface of the above-named liquids."

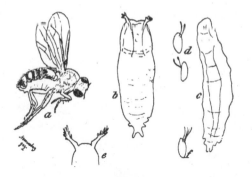

Drosophila fenestrarum, little vinegar fly.
a) male insect, b) pupa, c) larva, d) egg with 2 suction pads, seen from different angles, e) Drosophila funebris, large vinegar fly: upper end of the pupa with both spiracle tubes, f) eggs with 4 suction pads (15 x)

(Ref.: Henneberg, Handbuch der Gärungsbakteriologie, 2. Band, 1926, Verlag Paul Parey, Berlin & Hamburg.)

Control of vinegar flies

You can hardly completely avoid tiny vinegar flies buzzing around the fermentation container now and then. They don't do any harm by doing so. What you must absolutely avoid, however, is letting the flies get right inside the container and laying their eggs there, from which the unappetizing maggots begin to hatch and then crawl around the surface of the culture. If the following rules are observed, the battle against vinegar flies is in most cases already won:

1. You must cover the container with a cloth, a piece of muslin, a single layer peeled from a paper handkerchief, or anything similar which will let the air through but has no opening large enough to allow the tiny flies to creep through. The openings in net curtain material are often too large.

2. In addition – and this is very important! – the cloth must be firmly secured with a rubber band or a piece of string, so that there is no possibility of the flies getting through between the cloth and the side of the container.

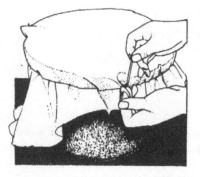

Control of vinegar flies: the cloth covering the container must be firmly secured with a rubber band or a piece of string.

You can defend yourself against swarms of tiny flies getting out of hand around the outside of the fermentation container by hanging up a strip of sticky fly-paper. Henneberg suggests (p. 357) "setting up bottle-traps. Narrow-necked bottles half filled with beer, vinegar or wine are just right for this. Care must be taken, however, that the acetic bacteria or film-forming yeasts do not build up a skin which covers the liquid completely, otherwise you won't achieve your goal. The liquid in the bottle-trap must therefore either be very acid indeed to begin with, or must be frequently renewed."

The best way to fight the vinegar flies to make a fly trap. This method is very good and effective: Just put some kombucha tea into a small wine or other glass. Additionally, pour some drops of dish detergent into the tea. The little critters can't resist the temptation to take a little swim. The flies sink to the bottom and drown. That is because there is no longer any surface tension on the liquid. It works great!

A further simple, but very effective way of controlling vinegar flies has been "invented" by my wife, and employed with great success: you take the vacuum-cleaner, remove the brush attachments etc., and simply hoover the pests away. When the flies have settled on the cloth covering the container and are savoring the heavenly kombucha smell, up you come with the vacuum-cleaner, hold the nozzle just above the cloth, and – whoosh – all the flies get sucked up the tube. The powerful suction can even catch them on the wing. Do that a few times a day, and you'll soon be left in peace.

Temporary suspension

Temporary suspension of kombucha production

A frequently heard question is: "I'm going away on holiday. What should I do with my kombucha culture during this time?" Let's ask Prof. Henneberg (1926). On page 379 of his Handbuch der Gärungsbakteriologie he gives this advice: "Should the production of kombucha be suspended for some time, a larger quantity of the beverage than usual should be left in the container, and the latter kept as cool as possible. In this way, the culture will remain viable for 3–4 weeks. Before using the culture again, the remaining very sour kombucha liquid should be poured off, and like any kombucha beverage that has accidentally become too sour, it can be used as table vinegar."

I absolutely agree with Prof. Henneberg, from whose books I have learned a great deal. From my own experience, however, I consider the period of 3–4 weeks mentioned by him to be too low an estimate. When kept cool, e.g. in a cellar with a temperature of 8-10° Celsius (50° Fahrenheit), the culture remains viable for months. I heard of a lady who, contrary to her husband's wishes, did not want to produce any more kombucha. She left the culture unheeded in the cellar, in the hopes that it would die. But the culture wouldn't oblige. Because her husband was so sorry that his wife wouldn't brew any more kombucha, she brought the culture back into the living area again after a few months and made a fresh attempt at brewing the beverage – and it worked.

In case you should have to leave the culture alone for a longer period of time, I recommend the following method, which causes no harm: shortly before your departure, place the culture in an open container with freshly made tea with sugar in it, with the usual addition of a proportion of ready-fermented beverage. Cover this container with a piece of muslin and stand it in a fairly cool place. e.g. on a clean shelf in the cellar. The activity of the culture slows down considerably because of the low temperature, but it doesn't die. You can leave it there for weeks. The culture can then begin working again at the same time as you do.

We occasionally also hear the advice to put the culture in a screw-top jar, fill it up with some ready-fermented kombucha, and put the sealed jar in the fridge. I consider it unnecessary to keep the fridge on just for the sake of the kombucha culture when one is absent for a longer period of time, when keeping it in a cool cellar works just as well. Besides, the culture takes longer to get going again after being kept in the fridge than when it has been kept in the cellar. Its viability does not sink to zero in the cellar, where the temperature is not so low. In the fridge, where it has to do without oxygen at 4° Celsius (39° Fahrenheit), the microorganisms will virtually completely cease their vital functions, and after a change in circumstances will react with a more or less marked phase of delayed activity.

Deep-freezing the kombucha culture

We are also often advised to deep-freeze the culture in the freezer during a break in production, together with a little of the ready-fermented beverage. To do this, the culture can be heat-sealed into a freezer bag or else put into a screw-top jar. When using screw-top jars, they should be left open at first so that they won't burst, and the lids only screwed on tight once the culture has been shock-frozen. The lids should be removed again before thawing, so that a vacuum does not form above the liquid.

Prof. Dittrich (1975, p. 70) writes about the influence of cold on the general development of microorganisms: "Compared with heat, it is virtually ineffectual. Reproduction is certainly very much slowed down by low temperatures, but death by freezing is hardly possible. This is of course in line with natural conditions, for whereas boiling heat hardly ever occurs, freezing of the substrate containing bacteria (e.g. earth) for months on end is the rule, even in our latitudes."

Prof. Henneberg (1926, Vol. 1, p. 6) confirms this: "In general, cold does not kill fungi. Bacteria, yeasts, mold spores can remain viable in ice for a long time. Even a temperature of -113 °C does not kill yeasts."

In my opinion, one has to be careful when freezing the culture that it does not suffer any damage due to the freezing process. If the temperature sinks so slowly during freezing that the culture remains for a very long time in the critical zone of 0 °C to -5 °C, this can damage it. This temperature range is critical because long sharp ice crystals slowly form during this time, and they destroy the cell walls. Crystals need time to grow. If they are not given this time, they cannot form. So it all depends on the culture being frozen to sleep very quickly – if possible, shock-frozen. It may therefore be advisable to turn on the fast freeze equipment or flick the super-frost switch and get the temperature right down ready before you put the culture in. Because of the speed of freezing and the intense cold, the critical zone of low temperature is passed through so quickly that large ice-crystals with their dangerous sharp edges and points cannot form. Rather, only small crystals develop which cannot injure the cell walls and the structure of the culture.

When thawing out the culture, the block of ice should be laid in fresh nutrient solution. In my experiments with frozen kombucha cultures, I have observed the following (the cultures were frozen from 8 days to 3 months):

At first, the cultures lay as if dead on the bottom of the fermentation container, and I thought they had frozen to death. Then little bubbles gradually began to rise – a sign that the yeasts were beginning to work and that carbonic acid was being produced. Only after some delay – about 14 days after thawing out the culture – could I observe a thin skin beginning to form on the surface of the tea. This told me that now the bacteria had taken up their production of cellulose, from which the skin is formed. After a little while a beautiful culture had formed again, although it seemed to me to be rather more jelly-like than usual. These processes happened much more quickly in control glasses.

For a long time, I could not explain the reason for this delayed development, and wondered whether some of the microorganisms had not been destroyed or damaged by the freezing process after all, and the remaining bacteria and yeasts must first build themselves up again. Then, I came across the following statement in Dr. Helga Schröder's book "Mikrobiologisches Praktikum" (Microbiological Practice – 1975), which could account for my observations: "If a nutrient solution is inoculated with bacteria, then growth does not begin in the 'typical' exponential way, but goes through a more or less marked phase of delay. This initial phase is called the latent period. The length of time it takes Is influenced among other things by the age of the inoculum (Note: = the substance which is added; old cells go through a long latent period) and by the composition of the milieu (when the composition of the nutrient solution in which the inoculum is cultivated and the one which is to be inoculated is the same, the latent period is shortened)."

The above-mentioned exponential growth means the phase during which the bacteria divide so quickly and so well that at certain intervals a doubling of the number of organisms takes place: one bacterium divides, and two cells are formed. They grow and divide in their turn, so that after the second division there are four cells. The number of cells is therefore doubled at every division. This system of constant doubling causes the quickest growth and in all cultures only lasts for a short time. We should otherwise soon be up to the ears in kombucha culture.

I suspect that the microorganisms need the long starting phase, as explained above, because of the complete contrast of the change in their living conditions. This should be understood, and concessions made for the culture if you think it should be frozen. Some people have even thrown the culture away because they thought it was dead after they had thawed it out.

Drying the culture

As a further possibility of keeping the culture inactive for a long time (e.g. during a long world trip), it should be mentioned that it is also possible to dry it. It then looks like a tough brownish leathery skin. When this skin is put into a nutrient solution, it swells, and the microorganisms begin to reproduce again. There is the danger, however, that depending on environmental conditions during the drying process, wild yeasts etc. present in the atmosphere might settle on the culture.

Incidentally, the tough dried skin has also been used for the production of imitation leather. Layers of kombucha culture which had grown imperfect concentric formation were tanned and then worked into kid gloves by the Auer Company (Lindner, 1913 and Harms, 1927).

Lakowitz (1928) also writes that during the war successful attempts were made to manufacture balloon envelopes from xylinum skin cultivated on a large scale.

Valentin (1928) devised a special method of producing a dried preparation. He cut up the culture and mixed it with chopped rosehip skins and dried this mixture at 30° C. With 10 g of this mixture per liter of nutrient solution he was able to make a good kombucha beverage even after one year.

Part 12

Personal experience

Testimonials

During my work on kombucha, I have received a good many reports from enthusiastic kombucha fans. In this enlarged third edition, and at the request of several readers, I shall let some of these kombucha-drinking correspondents speak for themselves. Copies of all reports printed below are held by the publishers. Like the articles mentioned above, the personal reports are also remarkable for the broad range of complaints for which people say they have received help. As I see it, this can be explained by the fact that the effect of kombucha is not aimed at any one specific organ, but by stabilizing the metabolism and by the detoxifying effect of the glucuronic acid in particular, it has a positive influence on the system as a whole. This then becomes apparent in many people by an increase in endogenic resistance to the harmful substances and environmental pollution bombarding us from every side, by a resuscitation of the damaged cells in the body, and by a restoration and consolidation of well-being. But let's allow a few heartening letters to speak for themselves.

Frau T. S. from P., Germany, writes:
"I've had it (the kombucha culture) for six months now, and my health is improving all the time. Briefly, I feel great. I also passed it on to friends who are also very happy with it and have been cured of rheumatic pains and liver complaints, for example, (...) I wouldn't like to have to give up drinking the beverage."

Herr A. H. from A., Germany, relates:
"A year ago I had to go to the doctor on account of my stomach pains. Tablets did not help me. Then by chance I happened to get some kombucha, and drink 2 glasses a day of it. It's only seldom that I feel any stomach pains now. So I presume the tea helped me."

Herr A. M. from B., Switzerland, had the following experience:
"I suffered for years from a lot of phlegm in the throat and could never get rid of it. It was particularly bad at bed-time. When I lay down, the phlegm completely blocked my throat, and despite all my efforts I couldn't get rid of it. That has improved since I've been drinking kombucha; the phlegm gets neutralized. (...) My wife had an injury to her right leg, and that gave rise to an infection with thrombophlebitis. The doctor wanted to send her to hospital, but I didn't want her to go. And with prayer and kombucha her leg healed up beautifully after a week. She also had less pain than is usual with this complaint."

Six month later Herr A.M. wrote again:
"And now I should like to tell you something else that I've noticed since we've been drinking kombucha. When I was about 16 years old and an apprentice blacksmith and wainwright, I drilled a hole through my left thumbnail while boring some holes, and ever since then it wasn't normal. It curved downwards. And now (Note: Herr A. M. is now 74 years old) I see that the nail is almost normal again. And 10 years ago I had a coronary heart operation (by-pass), and several lumps had formed on the scar which have also now disappeared. My wife had corns on her toes, and since I've been dabbing them with a wad of cotton wool soaked in kombucha, they've disappeared."

Frau J. S. from L., Germany, wrote two letters:
"Kombucha is the one and only remedy which helps my susceptibility to infection. Herbal remedies, homeopathic preparations, enzyme therapy, symbiotic control, treatment with my own blood, all

intended among other things to increase resistance, did not achieve the desired result. Besides this, I can ward off migraine attacks with kombucha. In my case, the migraines seem primarily to have a hormonal cause, as they mostly occur during menstruation. My chronic stomach and bowel trouble did actually improve after the symbiotic control treatment, but under greater pressure and in spring and autumn I still ended up with gastritis. With kombucha I can take a wholefood diet, which I'd already switched over to in the 70's. I don't need to do any more roll cures. My rheumatic pains (rheumatism of the soft tissues) have become noticeably less since taking the miracle drink. Earlier on I could only cope with the pain by taking enzymes. Now I only rarely have to reach for the 'Wobenzym'. (...) My husband feels physical and mental capacities have improved since taking kombucha. His blood pressure has returned to normal. He used to suffer from hypotonia. (...) A brother-in-law of mine seems not to be so depressive after drinking kombucha. He used to spend most of the day in bed. We couldn't believe our eyes when we saw that thanks to kombucha he'd painted all the windows of his house."

And now a few lines from Frau J. S.'s second letter:
"In connection with the weak resistance I've acquired over the years, I began to get cystitis and bronchitis at intervals that were much too close together. The athlete's foot between my toes also wouldn't go away. My bronchial tubes still give me a bit of bother in wet weather, but up till now I've been spared the tiresome cystitis. Fortunately, the athlete's foot has also departed. Incidentally, I can now at last continue with the symbiotic control treatment which has been dragging on since as far back as 1986, as without kombucha I frequently used to react to the vaccine injections with infections. (...) I think I shan't give up the 'miraculous jelly-fish' and I'll even increase the dosage. As I had a fit of the shivers etc. just now, I drank twice as much of the beverage. After drinking it, you always get this nice warm feeling and begin to perspire slightly, like when you've taken 'Echinacea' or any other immune stimulant. Proof that

one's resistance is beginning to work! (...) I'm very pleased that at nearly 40 I've at last found the remedy in KOMBUCHA, and can now face the future confidently and fearlessly."

Frau R. W. from L., Netherlands, writes:
"A great many people have been cured of the greatest variety of metabolic diseases by kombucha. In our tiny country one can now even speak of a kind of kombucha "revolution". GPs and specialists are often speechless at the relatively quick healing through kombucha, even in cases where they could achieve nothing for years and even decades with other remedies. (...) Some rheumatism patients told us that through kombucha they could do away with wheelchairs or crutches. Most reports tell of the healing of intestinal complaints, high blood pressure and rheumatic pains. Many people can sleep well again, thanks to kombucha. Healthy people experience an increase in energy. Athletes are absolutely delighted. Sometimes we ourselves can hardly believe reports.
But we know that kombucha has wide and far-reaching effects, cleansing and revitalizing. And then of course one feels better."

Frau L. B. from G. writes:
"I've felt much better since drinking kombucha. I've no more spots, my hair is much nicer, I was going gray, but all the gray hairs have vanished now. Menstruation is much more regular and less painful."

Herr L. Z. from D. writes:
"I'll gladly pass on to you my experiences with KOMBUCHA.
Until recently I was always having problems with my blood fat. The levels were always too high and normal levels could only be achieved by means of tablets. My attention was drawn to KOMBUCHA, and instead of the tablets I used only this beverage. The result was that normal levels could be maintained, thanks to KOMBUCHA. In addition, I also feel in general much better."

Frau H. S. from A. writes:

"I should like to thank you very much for the successful cure I've had by drinking your kombucha tea. For this success borders on the miraculous. Two years ago I had a complete hysterectomy due to carcinoma (cancer) or the womb. But after four months, a further operation was necessary. Following that I had thirty radiation treatments. But the result was that I was having up to eight bowel movements a day. All this without receiving any medication form the doctor. At that time, I happened quite by chance to read about kombucha tea." Frau S. says that she then got herself some kombucha and colibiogen etc., and then she goes on: "And what happened? The bowel movements returned to the normal two a day. During this time, I had to go into hospital for a check-up every two months. Then I learned from my doctor that the last two cancer smear tests were negative. The result amazed my doctor and the hospital doctors, as I had had no medication. I put it all down to the kombucha tea and the colibiogen etc. Therefore I thank you once again for this marvelous remedy, that hopefully will also help other women."

Herr O. H. from St. G. writes:

"I should like to tell you that I am very pleased with your kombucha cure. I followed the course for the purpose of purifying the system and in order to get rid of springtime lethargy. The course has helped me in every respect. I fell fit again."

S. K. from N. writes:

"I should like to tell you that I'm quite convinced about kombucha tea. I always used to be very tired in the evenings. Since I've been taking kombucha, that's all changed. I have much more energy again. It's really good stuff."

Frau T. v. K. from R. writes:

"I'm most enthusiastic about kombucha, as my digestion has returned to normal through using it. What a pity I didn't know about kombucha sooner."

15-year-old M. P. from K., Netherlands, sent an account entitled
"My good experience with kombucha:

The misery began when I was 10 years old, and it lasted for 4 ½ years. At first the itching began in my arms, and I scratched them till they bled, especially in bed at night. (...) After 6 weeks I then eventually went to the doctor. I was given a course of penicillin and ointment, because one arm was all inflamed from scratching. This lasted for about 1 ½ years. I kept on getting more ointment, one lot after the other, and it was the same with the penicillin. – Then I reached the point where things couldn't go on like that any more. I had to go to hospital for specialist treatment. The doctor talked about some intestinal bacteria which was the cause of the trouble.

Then I was given yet more medicine, which made me feel as if I was numb the whole time. But the itching remained. (...)

But now my mother's been making kombucha tea for the past six months. I began drinking it right away, and after only one week the itching had gone. I feel as if I've been born again. Even the scars are hardly visible any more. I'd like to tell everyone 'Stop taking medicine, and drink kombucha'."

Frau M. W. from V., Netherlands
has written an account that was published as a reader's letter in "Op Zoek", the magazine of the "Netherlands Multiple Sclerosis Foundation" (No. 141, February 1990).

"I've been suffering from multiple sclerosis since 1982. I've now had good results with kombucha. This has a detoxifying effect on the body. I began drinking the tea in 1989. At that time, I could only go a few meters outside the house, leaning heavily on two sticks, and my condition was getting visibly worse. Now I can get out again for about 20 minutes, without sticks, and I'm not tired any more. The result of a medical check-up was the renewal of the certificate of ability to hold a normal driving license. I'm even going to try a little skiing again this year. With a kombucha culture you can prepare your own natural remedy all your life long. I hope this account will contribute towards other people experiencing an improvement in their state of health through kombucha."

Frau H. Z. from H. writes:
"I've been cultivating a kombucha culture in our house for the past year, a task which gives me great pleasure. My husband drank only one glass of kombucha a day, and within 6-7 weeks he was free of rheumatism in both shoulders."

Professor J.S. from M.S., California, reports:
"I would like to share my experience with kombucha. In April 1994, bone cancer flared up and my right elbow started to dissolve. I could hardly use my right hand! The pain became almost unbearable. I could not sleep at nights. I could hardly walk. Nothing was of any help to improve my condition. I was ready to die. By the end part of July, my apartment manager gave me a pancake shaped mushroom. I started drinking the fermented mushroom tea, one cupful per day. In less than three weeks my elbow healed! Ever since I feel alive again, and I do have a lot of energy! I am not tired at all! What a bliss to have such a feeling. I am alive and well and full of hope! Thank you Günther W. Frank. ......Since then I have introduced the kombucha mushroom to many of my friends. From Hawaii to Alaska, Nevada, England, Hungary and all over in California. Every one gave a positive response. I would like to express my humble thanks for your tireless and thankless work that you have given to many of us who needlessly suffered the conventional medical treatment."

Documentary evidence
An amazing story from Russia

The following article was written by a man who studied medicine at the Lomonosov University in Moscow and the Military Academy in Leningrad from 1946 to 1954. He has emigrated since then, and now lives in the Federal Republic of Germany. Name and address are known to me, but the author wishes them not to be published. I should like to express my thanks to him for permitting me to print this interesting account of what happened behind the scenes.

Regardless of the Reagan intrigue, the Soviet experience is part of the large body of documentary evidence that the beverage made from kombucha fermentation of tea and sugar is, indeed, a dramatic immune system booster and body detoxifier. In our world and in our present time, our bodies surely need plenty of both – immune boosting and detoxification. This is essentially why I am so excited about the prospects of kombucha and why I will strive to spread the word as widely as possible.

KOMBUCHA

From the history of medicine in the USSR. – Episode from 1951 to 1953 and how the USA has profited by it since 1983. – Background to the breaking off of a promising research project on cancer therapy in the Soviet Union.

The Soviet scientists finally solved riddle of the cancer free population – Tea Kvass

After the great national war (1941-1945), the number of cancer cases in the Soviet Union, as in other lands, increased by leaps and bounds from year to year. At the beginning of 195, the Russian Academy of Sciences and the Central Oncological Research Institute in Moscow decided, among other important research measures, to analyze minutely the statistical data on the varying frequency of cancer cases in the individual regions, districts and cities of the USSR.

In doing so, the habits and environmental conditions of the populations in the districts where there were particularly few cases of cancer were to be investigated in especially close detail.

In this way – you might say almost criminologically – it was hoped to reach new discoveries in the field of pathogenesis and if possible succeed in finding an effective cure for cancer.

Conspicuous in this respect were the districts of Ssolikamsk and Beresniki in the region of Perm on the Kama in the central western Urals. **There were hardly any cases of cancer** here and then only in people who had just moved there.

The environmental conditions were no better here than in the old industrial areas. In the Ssolikamsk and Beresniki districts there was new and continually expanding industry which on account of its pollution (potassium, lead, mercury and asbestos mines and the dangerous processing works connected with them) was very much more dangerous than the old industrial areas in other parts of the Soviet Union.

Although the population density was considerably less, the pollution was in comparison considerably more dangerous. The trees were dying and so were the fish in the Kama.

Two Exploration teams of 10 scientists each, plus associated personnel, were set up. Dr. Molodyev headed the team in the Ssolikamsk district, and Dr. Grigoriev the team in Beresniki.

The techniques used in the exploration, which were very extensive and lengthy, need not be described in detail here.

Among other things explored by the teams were: origin of the population, ethnic differences, dwelling and living conditions, eating, drinking and sleeping habits, as well as leisure activities, age groups, and much more besides.

On no point did these innumerable factors, which were further subdivided, show any substantial difference to the populations in other areas of the USSR.

The laboratory measurements of the pollution and its effects on the earth, water, fauna and flora gave extremely unfavorable results.

If these unfavorable results had not intensified the contradiction to the fact that in spite of them there were hardly any cancer cases here, the investigations would probably have been long since broken off. Nevertheless, the long investigation revealed nothing of importance.

The only thing that stood out was that in spite of a comparatively higher consumption of alcohol and nicotine, the work morale was considerably better than in other areas of the USSR. Non-payment of social security contributions due to illness were considerably fewer. Drunken offenses were extremely rare. In spite of higher alcohol consumption, drunkenness was virtually unknown. It looked as if the people here could take more alcohol. The norms for work and production were being constantly and genuinely exceeded. The general mood of the population was on the whole high. Explanations for all these phenomena were however not at first forthcoming. There seemed to be little prospect of finding an explanation for them.

Tea wine the old Babushka said
One warm summer's day, the team leader Dr. Molodyev personally visited the dwelling of one of the families to be questioned. The wife and husband were out at work; the children were at kindergarten or play school. Only an old babushka was there, doing the housework. She helped several other related families as well in this way, which is why she couldn't look after the grandchildren at the same time.

The old babushka offered Dr. Molodyev refreshment, as the day was particularly hot, and he accepted gratefully. The beverage, which was unknown to Dr. Molodyev, he found pleasant, refreshing and tasty. When he inquired what sort of a drink it was, the old lady told him it was called "tea kvass."

Dr. Molodyev was astonished. He only knew of kvass which was fermented from bread. On inquiry, the old lady explained that "tea kvass" was not made from bread but from sweetened tea which was fermented by means of the "tea fungus" or "tea sponge." When the old babushka saw that Dr. M. had difficulty in understanding this, she showed him about 10 big stoneware jars which were standing side by side on shelves in a small neighboring room and which had muslin or linen cloths tied down over them. She uncovered one of the jars. It smelled strongly of fermentation. On the top floated a large round gray-brown jelly-like thing, flat as a pancake, which looked almost like a jelly-fish. "Not exactly appetizing", said Dr. M. "But very healthy for all that, easy to digest, and what's more, free", retorted the old lady.

Spongy thing looked ugly, but drink was tasty
She then described in precise detail for Dr. M. the method of preparing it: into the stoneware jar is poured 3-5 liters of warm black tea (1 teaspoonful of tea to 1 liter of water), sweetened with 100 to 150 grams of sugar per liter. While the tea is still lukewarm, a 'fungus' or an offshoot of one is placed on top, after a cup of ready-fermented tea kvass has been added. Then a linen or muslin cloth is bound over the jar. After standing for 10 to 12 days at 20 to 30 degrees C, the new tea kvass or "tea wine" is ready.

Of course, the culture propagates itself from time to time by a cylindrical binary fission. However, using a sharp blade, three or four kopeck-sized pieces of culture (about the size of a 1 Euro) can be cut from the edge of the main culture, like a gear wheel, and placed in small glass jars (150 ml) on black tea and kombucha beverage (in the ratio 1:1), sweetened as above. After three or four days new cultures will have grown, and they can replaced right away on 2 liters of tea plus kombucha beverage.

The Czar: "Give this wine to the people"
The old lady must surely have told him that there wasn't a family in the whole of the Ssolikamsk region that didn't brew and drink "tea wine". It had been so for many hundreds of years. It was said that learned travelers had brought it with them from China long ago. The Chinese had obtained it from the Japanese. The scholars had presented the Czar with this ferment with which one could make

wine out of tea. After a while the Czar remarked that this "wine" was no longer to his taste. He commanded it to be given to the people, with the comment that now everyone could make wonderful wine from tea. The little moujiks would stop being so covetous, and they wouldn't get drunk on this "wine" either.

By a similar strange coincidence, the team under Dr. Grigoriev in Berezniki also stumbled on this otherwise almost unknown tea ferment during their research. Long and thorough investigation proved that in both regions there was hardly a household which did not possess the "tea fungus", produce this strange "tea wine", and consume it in large quantities.

Here was a cheap and beneficial folk beverage. Even alcoholics drank large quantities of it before, during and after drinking alcohol. The remarkable thing about this was that after consuming large quantities of alcohol, drinkers showed hardly any signs of inebriation. Drunken offenses and accidents – either on the roads or at work – caused as a result of consuming alcohol, were extremely rare.

The consumption of alcohol and tobacco was rather higher in the areas investigated than in other regions of the USSR.

The Moscow Central Bacteriological Institute

Now came the scientific evaluation of the results of the investigation. This was made more difficult because nobody in either team was in a position to classify of define the sinister "tea fungus" with scientific exactitude. The Moscow Central Bacteriological Institute was able to help fairly quickly. Using color photos and samples, it was categorically established that they were dealing with the little-known KOMBUCHA.

Kombucha is the Japanese "tea sponge" or "tea fungus", which is a jelly-like mass formed of Bacterium xylinum and netlike deposits of yeast cells of the genus Saccharomyces. To this symbiosis also belong: Saccharomyces ludwigii, Saccharomyces of the apiculatus types, Bacterium xylinoides, Bacterium gluconicum, Schizosaccharomyces pombe, Acetobacter ketogenum, Torula types, Pichia fermentans and other yeasts.

It was also known that this kombucha was used in some parts of the Soviet Union to prepare a cider-like beverage called "tea kvass".

But the Central Bacteriological Institute in Moscow did not know much more about kombucha than this. They relied mainly on the manual written by the German W. HENNEBERG, "Handbuch der Gärungsbakteriologie", Vol. 2, 1926.

But the German manual did not say anything about the biochemical functions of the kombucha symbiosis either. So now the Central Biological and Biochemical Institute in Moscow was consulted.

Kombucha is not a mushroom or fungus

We now know that the so-called "kombucha tea fungus" is not a fungus but a lichen. Kombucha is a symbiosis of yeast cells and bacteria, a fungal lichen membrane which does not reproduce my means of spores – like a fungus – but by budding. (Note by G. W. Frank: I hope the author of this article will forgive me, but I do not agree with the classification of kombucha as a lichen. A lichen is a symbiosis of algae and fungi, and requires light as a source of energy to build up chlorophyll by photosynthesis, a typical feature of algae. kombucha on the other hand flourishes even in the dark, precisely because it contains no algae components. a typical feature of lichens.)

Kombucha turns the tea into a sea of health giving acids and nutrients

Detailed investigation revealed that kombucha, apart from other not easily definable substances possessing an antibiotic effect, produces GLUCURONIC ACID in particular, vitamins B1, B2, B3, B6, B12 as well as folic acid and dextrogyral, i.e. L-LACTIC ACID (+).

The GLUCURONIC ACID and the dextrogyral L-LACTIC ACID (+) were of prime interest here. A healthy liver produces sufficient quantities of GLUCURONIC ACID, which, as yet, can hardly be produced synthetically. It binds our own metabolic toxins and exogenous environmental pollutants which have entered the body and are then transferred via the gallbladder into the intestines and via the kidneys into the urine. Toxins bound by the glucuronic acid cannot be reabsorbed by the intestines or the urinary system. Glucuronic acid consequently has an extraordinarily important detoxifying function. A healthy body can produce it in sufficient quantities in the liver under normal circumstances, ensuring in general and adequate detoxification of the system. It becomes critical when the environment contains excessive amounts of freely circulating toxic substances or when excessive amounts of endogenic metabolic toxins accumulate in the body.

Do people today have healthy livers? Not really! So they need kombucha

The gradually and increasingly weakened liver cannot manage to produce sufficient glucuronic acid any more. In a situation where excessive amounts of endogenic and environmental toxins are present, the development of cancer and other diseases is fostered. Above all, the endogenic resistance system (RES) breaks down.

Besides this, it is of great significance that GLUCURONIC ACID in conjugated form is the building block of the very important polysaccharides such as hyaluronic acid (ground substance of connective tissue), chondroitin-sulphuric acid (ground substance of cartilage) mucoitin-sulphuric acid (building block of the stomach lining and the vitreous humor of the eye) and heparin.

So it is not surprising that kombucha is USNIC ACID, normally obtained from lichen. It has a strongly antibacterial effect, and can even partly inactivate viruses. USNIC ACID is a dibenzofurane derivative.

Kombucha produces the good (+) lactic acid

L-LACTIC ACID (+) (dextrogyral) is almost never present in the connective tissue of cancer patients. So long as it is predominantly present in tissue, cancer cannot develop. It is interesting to note here that a pH value of 7.56 is exceeded in cancer patients. Organisms which are free from cancer (and also free from precancers) show pH values of under 7.5. A deficiency of L-LACTIC ACID (+) (dextrogyral) in the diet leads to failure of cell respiration, fermentation during the breakdown of sugar, and the build-up of DL-lactic acid in the tissue. Mixtures of both lactic acids (levogyral (-) and dextrogyral (+), i.e. D and L-lactic acid) in equal amounts, whose directions mutually cancel each other out, are called racemates. These racemates promote the development of cancer, and even make it possible in the first place.

Plenty of food containing dextrogyral, i.e. L-lactic acid, manual labor, muscle-training, saunas, etc., besides the elimination of waste products, enables the body to get rid of this lactic acid and thus regulates the pH value of the blood and helps to lower it. Serological tests of the blood in the veins have shown that the kombucha beverage shifts the pH value noticeably towards the acid side.

That should give you the broad outline of our chief interest in kombucha.

Detailed urine tests showed that after drinking kombucha, the urine of patients who had never drunk before contained considerable traces of environmental toxins (such as lead, mercury, benzol, caesium, etc.). It was thus determined that the beverage was completely free from these substances.

I shall have to tell Comrade Stalin about this

Prof. Vinogradov, member of the Academy of Sciences of the USSR, who was also Stalin's personal physician, ordered a series of further medical and pharmacological tests using kombucha. Rumors of a future miracle cure for cancer reached the ears of the Minister of the Interior and Chief of Secret Service, L. P. Beria, who had himself taken on a guided tour of the laboratories of the various research institutes that were now busy testing kombucha, and had everything explained to him in minute detail.

When Beria heard how they had come across kombucha, he was jubilant. "That's the criminological investigation method of our KGB for you! You see? Science can learn from the KGB! But learning from the KGB means learning how to be victorious! – I shall have to tell Comrade Stalin about this. He just recently reproached me and said that we must work more efficiently, that is scientifically."

In this context, people began to talk about how Stalin's anxiety about the possibility of getting cancer was growing ever greater. He kept on having nightmares about dying of cancer. Added to this, there was a scientific treatise by Prof. Petrovsky, Principal of the Leningrad Institute for Parapsychology, who said that people very often die of the disease they've always dreamt about. Stalin had apparently read this treatise, and due to his "belief in science" was now so depressed, that something had to happen.

In view of this state of affairs and because harmful side effects could with certainty be ruled out, Stalin was pacified by treating him with the raw product of kombucha, the beverage itself, before a corresponding pharmaceutical preparation could be developed. Prof. Vinogradov made his decision in this respect dependent on the assent of a medical council. In the autumn of 1952, a council meeting of 12 doctors gave their assent. Beria gave the go-ahead. But he had given his consent without reckoning on both of his deputies, KGB Generals Ryumin and Ignatiev. Both had got wind of the affair and had likewise had themselves conducted round the laboratories, naturally not without listening to the relevant scientific explanations about it, but then however coming to different conclusions.

Ryumin and Ignatiev were pathologically ambitious. Each of them was trying to oust Beria and take over the office of Minister of the Interior and Chief of KGB for himself. As Stalin at this time had considerable antipathies towards the Jews, which had never previously been the case, they used the fact that Vinogradov and most of the members of the council of Stalin's personal physicians were Jews.

They hatched a very primitive but, nonetheless, mean and effective plot, by informing Stalin that Vinogradov and his "accomplices" had cultivated particularly dangerous "molds" in order to obtain poisons from them with which they intended to slowly and unobtrusively but surely poison him (Stalin).

The Trial of the Moscow Doctors

Stalin in his extremely morbid distrust gave Ryumin and Ignatiev full power – without any interference from Beria – to arrest Vinogradov and his followers and to prepare a trial. This affair became known as "The Trial of the Moscow Doctors" 1953.

Vinogradov and his team of doctors landed up in Moscow's Lubyanka prison. The research work on kombucha came to an abrupt end.

The Moscow examining magistrates and public prosecutors soon discovered new "crimes" and formulated them in the indictment: damaging the reputation of Soviet medicine and pharmacology by relapsing into pre-scientific nature healing. They had deliberately tried to use this to ridicule Soviet science in the eyes of the world. Scientifically made preparations could not be seriously set aside in favor of pre-scientific so-called "nature products", without appearing backward and ridiculous.

Vinogradov and the other members of the "council of personal physicians" were vindicated after Stalin's death, and Beria, Ryumin and Ignatiev sentenced to death and executed for these machinations, but as far as I know, the research work on kombucha was not taken up again.

The Soviet Research Committees justified the indictment in the following way:

Soviet science refuses to slavishly imitate or exploit natural processes. Soviet science must think and investigate in an independent and creatively productive way. One should not stick to simple natural processes and copy them. This would be unworthy of a Soviet scientist. The aim of Soviet medicine is to create an irrefutable theory of the pathogenesis of cancer and to develop from it steps towards and effective therapy of this disease. Soviet medicine must not demean itself by descending to a state of quackery infatuated with nature cures. The former method of healing by natural means is pre-scientific. One should not fall back into such a state.

Kombucha for prisoners

However, nobody was against experiments with KOMBUCHA going on – on the quiet – in prison hospitals and labor camps, with prisoners who had got cancer. Thank God, these experiments did no harm in any way, but on the contrary only did good.

A vast number of specialist books have been written on this subject. As witness to this, **Alexander Solzhenitzyn's works** can be mentioned here, particularly "Cancer Ward", "The Right Hand", his autobiographies, etc.

In them, he expounds in detail how he himself fell hopelessly ill in prison from stomach cancer with numerous metastases in the lungs, liver, bowel, etc., and how by a seeming miracle he was completely cured by kombucha, which was made with birch-leaf tea. He then describes in "Cancer Ward" how he was in a Moscow clinic for a check-up, lying in the same room as some high-up officials who were also suffering from cancer, and who would have given all they possessed in order to get hold of this "miracle cure".

A note is necessary her: KOMBUCHA is made with **birch-leaf tea** in those cases where the urinary system requires stimulation.

The toxins bound by the glucuronic acid can thus be eliminated from the body particularly quickly and effectively. However, it must not be forgotten that the tea solution in which the KOMBUCHA culture is to be placed must always contain some black tea. Without black tea the KOMBUCHA culture will not thrive, if at all.

It is a little known fact that Paracelsus fermented all the medicinal herbs one could think of with KOMBUCHA. These medicinal herbs fermented with KOMBUCHA were particularly effective.

How the USA derived benefit

In 1983 the media reported for the first time that the President of the United States, Ronald Reagan, was said to have cancer. Then at regular intervals, we heard continual reports of new metastases which had appeared and had to be removed from bowel, bladder and nose. He found it difficult to cope with the chemotherapy he had at first been given. Further metastases appeared. Famous doctors in the USA remembered the cancer therapy mentioned by Alexander N. Solzhenitzyn in his Autobiography and "Cancer Ward." He had been cured of cancer quickly, completely and without problems in Soviet hard labor camp hospitals.

References to the sinister "tea fungus", allegedly the cause of the cure, were followed up. A. N. Solzhenitzyn, who was living as an immigrant in the USA, was questioned on this matter. He was able to give important information. Some samples of the "Japanese tea fungus", also called "Kombucha", were procured at once from Japan.

Treatment using this beverage began. President Ronald Reagan drank a liter of kombucha daily. Since that time, there were no further reports about either his cancer or his metastases. The president continued to enjoy many happy and healthy years of a life. His death on the 5th of June 2004 was at the ripe old age of 93 years.

A final word:
Is health the most important thing?

"The main thing is to stay healthy!" – how often does this phrase crop up in our conversation? Is health the main thing? In the visitors' book of a guest-house in world-famous Marienbad (Sudetenland) a spa patient had written the following couplet as a memento:

"I go back home in happiness;
Here found I health and highest bliss"

The Berlin pastor Johannes Evangelista Gossner (1773-1858) read the entry and in answer wrote beneath:

"Not highest bliss, 'tis only half,
For blissful else were a healthy calf."

The reality of daily life confirms this. Many people are bursting with good health and yet live at odds with themselves and the world. On the other hand, there are some who have been suffering from some illness for years, often bed-ridden and unable to take a single step outside the house – and yet they are the happiest people alive. I'm thinking of that American girl called Joni Eareckson – paralyzed from the neck down. Since a bathing accident when she was seventeen years old, she has had to live in a wheelchair. And this same Joni describes herself as the happiest person on earth because Jesus has enriched her life. Through such witnesses to life as this, the oft heard and much quoted phrase "The main thing is to stay healthy" is open to question.

However important all these things may be, I do not want to end this book without making the following final remark: don't place the interests of the body above those of the soul. Don't let food and health became an obsession that takes up all your time and completely dominates your thoughts. Don't pay attention with hypochondriacal exactitude to every flicker of emotion and every slightest alteration in your bodily functions which lie within the limits of normal fluctuation.

We have a certain responsibility to keep our bodies in good health, as far as it lies within our power to do so, as a loan from God. Yet, we should also be warned against turning the body and its health into a cult object. Health, the preservation of health, and philosophies of health can become an ersatz religion which occupies all our thoughts and efforts, whereby to a certain extent our own body becomes idolized. How would it be if we were to take the following warning as a guideline:

> *"Do not give yourself over to sorrow,*
> *and do not afflict yourself deliberately.*
> *Gladness of heart is the life of man,*
> *and the rejoicing of a man is length of days.*
> *Delight your soul and comfort your heart,*
> *and remove sorrow far from you,*
> *for sorrow has destroyed many,*
> *and there is no profit in it."*
>
> Ecclesiasticus 30:21-24

Basically, in a form that can be understood by all, these verses contain aspects of the new integral scientific discipline of psychoneuroimmunology, which examines the influence of the spirit on the development and course of illness. In this field, which in a very short period of time has experienced and undreamt-of upswing, amazing parallels have been discovered between psyche, central nervous system and immune system. The connections mesh together in a complicated manner and represent a biological information processing system.

To prevent cancer and infections, a balance between psyche, central nervous system and endocrine system must exist in the immune system. The endocrine system is the inner information, control and regulation system of the hormone producing glands and organs.

A whole army of defense specialists in the body is constantly resisting invasive attempts of various disease germs. Whereas, the immune system was, until recently, regarded as a self-regulating system, the interrelationship of all physical systems was set, in comparison, by present day stress research and immune biology. Previous experiments have shown that the immune system is closely bound up with the brain and the psyche through an information system. Brain and psyche intervene as a spur or a brake in the resistance battles between the defense specialists (leukocytes, phagocytes, lymphocytes, granulocytes, macrophages, cytokines, killer-cells) and the disease invaders.

Through their connection with the central nervous system and the psyche, these immune cells in man are not immune from stress. Tests in the USA have shown that spiritual tension in the sense of distress, e.g. exam nerves, visits to the dentist, loss of near relatives, depression, pessimistic outlook etc. weakens the immune system. With the weakening of the immune system goes an increased susceptibility to various illnesses. References for psychoneuroimmunology: Schultz (1986), Uhlenbruck (1988), factum (1988).

Conversely, this discovery has a positive side to it: everything that produces relaxation, cheerfulness, peace and composure, draws in its wake a strengthening of the powers of resistance. What sound scientifically very complicated has long since been graphically and uncomplicatedly expressed in the vernacular in the following rule:

He who smiles thrice in the morn,
and at noonday does not frown,
and every evening sings aloud,
of 99 years shall be proud.

To be sure, even by following this recipe for which no doctor's prescription is necessary, not everyone will live to be 99. We must keep clearly in mind that it is a natural process that our bodies will in the end grow old and die. However much we lavish care and attention on our bodies, sooner or later death will occur. We should reflect on that and thereby become wiser. That is what is intended by the motto of several Catholic orders: "Memento mori!" (Bear death in mind) Or as we read in Psalm 90, verse 12: "Teach us to number our days aright, that we may gain a heart of wisdom." (NIV)

Not everyone would be happy with Berthold Brecht's observation that "You're all going to die like animals, and there's nothing to come after that!" In every human lives a natural desire for life, for perfect and everlasting life.

As we continue our journey towards physical, psychological and spiritual health, we should perhaps take a moment to consider that the time we have here is limited. It is just borrowed. The following vivid anecdote exemplifies this perfectly:

A tourist stays the night in a monastery. He is astonished by the spartan furnishing of the cells and asks a brother, "Where is your furniture?" The quick-witted monk asks back, "And where is yours?" "Mine?" replies the tourist rather confused. "But, I am just passing through here." "Exactly," answers the monk. "So are we."

Acknowledgments

I thank

- the numerous people who have contributed to the production of this book by their suggestions, information, advice, comments, procuring of books and articles, personal experiences, questions, discussion, criticism and encouragement.

I should especially like to thank

- Dr. M. O. Bruker, Lahnstein, for his suggestions and corrections of the discussion on the question of the sugar problem,
- Prof. Ludmilla Tatyevossovna Danielova, Yerevan, USSR, for her willingness to let me know about the results of her researches and for sending me her scientific articles,
- Herr H. J. Ehmke, Welver-Flerke, for translating some Russian articles on kombucha for me, as well as the correspondence arising therefrom, and for giving me much valuable advice and encouragement,
- Drs. V. and J. Köhler, for letting me know about their results with glucuronic acid, and for patiently explaining the interrelationship to me,
- Frau Ingeborg Oetinger, Öhringen, for her suggestions and assistance with the study of the acid/alkali problem,
- Herr Erich Rasche, engineer, Friesenheim, for his bio-electronic researches by the Vincent method, and his guidance in connection with water quality.
- Dr. Jürgen Reiss, Microbiological Institute Grahamhaus Studt KG, Bad Kreuznach, for sending me his own photos and allowing me to use illustrations, tables and extracts from the next of his article on the metabolic products of the kombucha culture,
- Herr Joseph Rosen, Bielefeld-Sennestadt, for assistance with proof-reading and for his advice and help,
- Frau Ingrid Schmidt, Bochum, for sending me her article on kombucha and for allowing me to publish her photomicrographs and photomacrographs,

- Prof. Eduard Stadelmann of the Department of Horticultural Science, University of Minnesota, for sending me the translation of the Russian articles and for helping me considerably by contributing further information,
- Prof. Ulf Stahl, Microbiological Research Institute, Technical University of Berlin. to whom I am much obliged for help in elaborating and understanding the microbiological relationships within the Kombucha culture,
- Miss Althea Tyndale, Cambridge University, for translating this book and for the pleasant and enjoyable work together, during which time she devoted herself wholeheartedly and creatively to the task,
- Frau Regine Weessies, Leiderdorp, Netherlands, for the open and fruitful exchange of thoughts and experiences, for her inspiration, and for her constant encouragement that I should write this book,
- the tea experts, tea firms, and the German Tea Office in Hamburg for all the informative leaflets and documents they sent me,
- the publishers and authors for permission to use illustrations and extracts from texts as well as a complete article in the section supplying documentary evidence,

- the publishing house of Ennsthaler in Steyr for publishing this book and for being patient with me until I could send them the manuscript,
- my wife, Rosemarie, and my children Christopher, Manuel, Mirjam and Simon, from whom great patience was often required as this book progressed, and who had to do without many family ventures during this time.

Bibliography

Publications which deal predominately with Kombucha or which in one or another are of significance for its description, treatment, assessment etc., are printed in bold type. This bibliography does not only contain the sources, that Günther W. Frank used for writing this book, but also articles that were published later

ABELE, Johann: Macht saure Nahrung krank? Der Naturarzt 109 (5/1987), 13 u. 16

ABELE, Johann: Teepilz Kombucha bei Diabetes? Der Naturarzt 110 (12/1988), 31

AHLHEIM, Karl-Heinz (Hrsg.): Schülerduden, die Biologie. 464 Seiten, Mannheim 1976

AINSWORTH, G. C.: Dictionary of the Fungi. 6. Auflage, Commomwealth Mycological Institute, Kew 1971

Anonymous: Die Heilkraft des Pilzes Kombucha, Diagnosen 8 (9/1986), 72-73

Anonymous: Fungojapon, Pharmazeutische Zentralhalle 70 (1929), 267

Anonymous: The Mushroom Culture. The Journal of Mushroom Cultivation # 16, October 1994. Pensacola, Florida 1994

Anonymous: Mit weinähnlichem Geschmack. Hamburger Abendblatt No. 137 of 15th June 1983, page 10

Anonymous: Teepilz Kombucha neu entdeckt. Informationen Naturheilverein Pforzheim, Nr. 11/87, 2

Anonymous: Kombucha. Politische Hintergrund-Informationen (Basel) 7, S. 286 (07.11.88) und 329 (31.12.88)

Anonymous: Blitzschnell schön mit Bio-Tee. Bild der Frau (Hamburg) Nr. 1 vom 02.01.1990, 22-23

Anonymous: Kennnen Sie Kombucha? Gesundes Leben (Eschwege) 67, Nr. 2/1990, 34

Anonymous: Kombucha als Fitmacher. Raum & Zeit (Wiesbaden) 9, Nr. 47, Sept/Okt. 1990, 39-40

Anonymous: Kombucha gegen Zipperlein. Tip der Woche (Heilbronn) vom 26.03.1990, 5

Anonymous: Endlich Schluß mit der Frühjahrsmüdigkeit. Bio spezial Nr. 2/1990 (April/Mai 1990), 42-43

Anonymous: Kombucha – fast ein neuer Zaubertrank. Strick & Schick (Bergisch Gladbach) Nr. 4 (April 1990), 26-27

Anonymous: Neue entdeckt: Kombucha – Chinesisches Hausmittel. Pforzheimer Zeitung Nr. 22, 21.04.1990, 55

Anonymous: Neues vom Kombucha-Teepilz. Waerland Monatshefte (Düsseldorf) 40, (7/8/1990), 16-22 (Nachdruck aus "Lebensschutz-Informationen" Vlotho)

Anonymous: Deshalb schützt Kombucha vor Umweltgiften. Bio Spezial (Tutzing) Nr. 3/1990 (Juni/Juli 1990), 62-63

Anonymous: Kombucha diätetisches Lebensmittel. Pharmazeutische Zeitung 135, Nr. 8 vom 22.02.1990, 51

Anonymous: Kombucha – das Geheimnis seiner heilsamen Wirkung. Bio spezial (Tutzing) Nr. 1/1990

(Febr./März 1990, 32-33)

Anonymous: Neues vom Teepilz Kombucha. Bio Spezial (Tutzing) Nr. 1/1991 (Februar/März 1991), 31

Anonymous: Kombucha-Tee – wie man's macht (Leserzuschrift). Gesundheits-Nachrichten (Teufen/Schweiz) 48 (2/1991, Februar 1991), 32

Anonymous: Teepilz und japanische Kristalle. Deine Gesundheit (Berlin) Nr. 1/91, 21

Anonymous: Der Kombuchapilz schützt sich selber. Sonnseitig leben (Zürich) 42, Nr. 226 (Juni/Juli 1991), 17

Anonymous: Pilze im Tee. Sonnseitig leben (Zürich) 42, Nr. 227 (Aug./Sept. 1991), 19

Anonymous ("thy"): Kombucha ist erfrischend und unschädlich. Hessische Allgemeine – Sonntagszeitung (Kassel) Nr. 24, 14. Juni 1992, 24

Anonymous: Trinken Sie sich fit. Sonderbeilage zu DIVA Nr. 67 (Mai 1997), Seite 2 Verlag Radda & Dressler Verlagsges.m.b.H., Davidgasse 79, 1100 Wien, Österreich

Anonymous: "Kombucha trinken – den Körper entgiften",

Neue Gesundheit (Klambt-Verlag GmbH & Cie. Baden-Baden) Nr. 3, März 1998, 24

Anonymous: Ein Pilz erobert Hollywood – Madonna & Co. schwören auf Kombucha. "freundin" (München) Nr. 18 vom 12. August 1998, Seite 16.

ARAUNER, E.: Der japanische Teepilz. Dtsch. Essigindustrie 33 (2/1929), 11-12

ARTZ, Neal E., Osman, Elizabeth M.: Biochemistry of Glucuronic Acid. New York, Academic Press. New York 1950

ALTHOFF, Nadeen: Wie aus Kombucha Natur Pur wurde. Raum und Zeit 13 (Nr. 71, Sept/Okt. 1994, Dietramszell), 68-71

AVILA, Jana: Der Pilz, der im Tee wächst. Schweizer Familie Nr. 7 (13. Februar 1997), Seite 50 (Auflage 232.000, erscheint wöchentlich)

BACH, H.-D.:Äußere Kennzeichen innerer Erkrankungen. 352 Seiten. 1989, Münster (Seite 332: "Andere setzen auf die Heilkraft des Teepilzes Kombucha")

BAcINSKAJA, A. A.: O rasprostranenii "cajnogo kwasa" i Bacterium xylinum Brown. zurnal Microbiologii (Petrograd) 1 (1914), 73-85 (Von der Verbreitung des "Teekwaß" und des Bacterium xylinum Brown)

BAENKLER, H.: Klinische Immunologie, Profil eines jungen Faches. cesra-Säule 50 (1988), 12-19

BALIS, Frans und Roos Van Hoof: Koemboecha of Kargasok – Eeuwenoud Levenselixir brengt opnieuw gezondheid (in niederländischer Sprache). 144 Seiten. 1991 Farma-Import, B-Beverlo-Beringen/Belgien

BARBANcIK, G. F.: cajnyj grib i ego lecebnye svojstva. Izdame Tret'e. Omsk: Omskoe oblast-noe kniznoe izdatel'stvo. 54 Seiten (Der Teepilz und seine therapeutischen Eigenschaften. Dritte Auflage). 1958

Bayerischer Rundfunk, Fernsehen Bayern 3, Bavaria – Magazin am Mittag: 31.Juli 1998, 12:02 bis 12:30 Uhr: Komboucha-Tee und seine Heilkraft

BAZAREWSKI, S.: Über den sogenannten "Wunderpilz" in den baltischen Provinzen. Correspondenzblatt Naturforscher-Verein, Riga 57, (1915), 61-69

BECK, U.: Wissenschaft und Sicherheit. Der Spiegel 43 (1988), 200-201

BEGUIN, M. H.: Gute Zähne dank vollwertigem Zucker, Separatdruck aus "Die Frauenschule" Nr. 11, 1978

BÉGUIN, Félix: Erfahrungen mit dem Teepilz Kombucha. Sonnseitig leben (Zürich) 41, Nr. 222 (Okt./Nov. 1990), 1517

BELITZ, H. D. u. W. GROSCH: Lehrbuch der Lebensmittelchemie. 2. Auflage, 799 Seiten, Springer, Berlin, 1985

BINDER, Franz u. Josef WAHLER: Zucker , nein danke. Heyne-TB-Verlag, München 1987

BING, M.: Heilwirkung des "Kombuchaschwammes". Umschau 32 (1928), 913-914

BING, M.: Der Symbiont Bacterium xylinum Schizosaccharomyces Pombe als Therapeutikum. Die medizinische Welt 2 (42), 1576-1577, (1928)

BING, M.: Zur Kombuchafrage. Die Umschau 33 (6), 118-119, (1929)

BIRKENBEIL, Helmut: Einführung in die praktische Mikrobiologie. 144 Seiten, Verlag Moritz Diesterweg, Frankfurt, 1983

BRAUDE, A.I., G.E. Vaisberg, T.I. Afanas'eva und N.I. Givental: A Study of the Stimulation of the Antibacterial Factors of the Body by Ciin. Antibiotics (Washington) 4. (3) 276-281

BRECHMANN, I. u. M. GRINEWITSCH: Die "Kerne" östlicher Rezepturen. Wissenschaft in der UdSSR (Moskau), Nr. 6/1988, 30-35 und 102

BROWN, A. J.: On an acetic Ferment which forms Cellulose. Journal of the Chemical Society (London) 49 (1886), 432-439

BRUKER, M. O.: Unser täglich Brot und der Fabrikzucker als Hauptursache für die modernen Zivilisationskrankheiten (Kleinschrift Nr. 1) emu-Verlags-GmbH, Lahnstein, o. J.

BRUKER, M. O.: Krank durch Zucker. Helfer, Schwabe, Bad Homburg 1981

BRUKER, M. O. u. I. GUTJAHR: Biologischer Ratgeber für Mutter und Kind. bioverlag gesundleben, Hopferau 1982

BRUKER, M. O.: Antwort auf Leseranfrage zu Kombucha. Der Naturarzt 108 (11/1986), 14

BRUKER, M. O.: Antwort auf Leseranfrage zu saurer Nahrung. Der Naturarzt 108 (11/1986), 14

BRUKER, M. O.: Honig-Verträglichkeit. Der Gesundheitsberater 11/1988, 18

BRUKER, M. O.: Antwort auf Leseranfrage "Wundermittel Kombucha?". Natur u. Heilen 65 (1988), 563

BRUKER, M. O.: Ärztlicher Rat aus ganzheitlicher Sicht. 449 Seiten, emu-Verlag, Lahnstein 1989

BRUKER, M.O.: Kombucha. Der Gesundheitsberater (Lahnstein) Nr. 4/1991 (April 1991), 12

BUSCHEK, Marcel: Uralter Jungbrunnen. Astro Venus Nr. 8/94 (München, August 1994), S. 38-41. München 1994

CARSTENS, V.: Hilfe aus der Natur meine Mittel gegen den Krebs. Quick Nr. 43/1987, 60-64

CBS (US television station): Evening News on December 14, 1994: Kombucha in Beverly Hills

CBS (US television station): This Morning on January 16, 1995: Consumer Report on Kombucha

CLARK, P. L.: How to live and eat for health. Chicago 1931

DAHL, Jürgen: Ein Glas Pilz ohne Schaum. Natur 7/1987, 73-74

DANIELOVA, L. T.: Bacteriostaticeskoe i bactericidnoe svojstvo nastoja "čajnogo griba". Trudy Erevanskogo zooveterinarnogo Instituta 11 (1949), 31-41 **(Die bakteriostatischen und bakteriziden Eigenschaften des Teepilz-Aufgusses)**

DANIELOVA, L. T.: K morfologii "čajnogo griba". Trudy Erevanskogo zooveterinarnogo Instituta 17 (1954), 201-216 **(Zur Morphologie des Teepilzes)**

DANIELOVA, L. T.: "čagnyj grib" Medusomyces Gisevii. Autoreferat Diss., predst. soisk. ucen. step. diktora veterinariyh. Moskva: Moskovskaja veterinarija akamedija, 36 Seiten, 1954 **(Der Teepilz Medusomyces Gisevii. Autoreferat der Diss. zur Erlangung des Doktortitels der Veterinärwissenschaften)**

DANIELOVA, L. T.: Biologičeskie osobennosti cajnogo griba. Trudy Erevanskogo zooveteri-narnogo Instituta 23 (1959), 159-164 **(Die biologischen Besonderheiten des Teepilzes)**

DANIELOVA, L. T. u. G. A. ŠAKARJAN: Teyi saki koultouran ew nra kiraroume, anasnapahoutyan mej. Erewan: gitoutyan glxavor varcoutyan hratarakcoutyoun. 160 Seiten, 1959 **(Die Kultur des Teepilzes und dessen Verwendung in der Viehzucht. Erewan: Verlag der Hauptverwaltung für Landwirtschaft)**122

DAVID, Wolfgang: Experimentelle Mikrobiologie, 4. Auflage, 142 Seiten, Quelle und Meyer, Heidelberg, 1981

DIETRICH, G. u. R. HUNDT, G. KOPPRASCH, G. KUMMER, K. LO-BECK, I. MEINCKE, R. STADE, H. THEUERKAUF: Wissensspeicher Biologie. 1. Auflage, 416 Seiten, Volk und Wissen Volkseigener Verlag, Berlin 1980

DINSLAGE, E. u. W. LUDORFF: Der "indische Teepilz". Zeitschrift für Untersuchung der Lebensmittel 53 (1927), 458-467

DITTRICH, H. H.: Bakterien, Hefen, Schimmelpilze. 5. Auflage, 87 Seiten, Kosmos-Verlag Franck, Stuttgart 1975

DUBOIS, J.-P.: Etats-Unis: un champignon dans la tête. Le Nouvel Observateur No. 15/96, pp. 92-93

ELMAU, H.: Bio-Elektronik Vincent. Erfahrungsheilkunde 34 (1985), 695-698

ENGLISCH, Otto: Krebs und seine biologische Bekämpfung. 2. Auflage, 213 Seiten, Intra-Ver-lag Kiel u. Dortmund 1981

ERMOL'EVA, Z. V. u. G. E. VAJSBERG u. T. I. AFANAS'EVA u. N. I. GIVENSTAL': O stimuljacii nekotoryh antibakterial'nyh faktorov v organizme žitvotnyh. Antibiotiki (Moskva) 3 (1958), (6), 46-50 (Über die Stimulierung bestimmter antibakterieller Faktoren im Tierorganismus)

ERMOL'EVA, Z. V.: Primenenie antibiotikov v medicine. In: (Herausgeber: Sovet narodnogo hozjajstva g. Moskva; Rcihc: Dostiženija nauki i tchnki) Primenenie antibiotikov v narodnom hozjajstve. Sokraščennaja stenogramma sovešcanija, sostojavšegosja 24-25 dakabrja 1957 g., S. 25-32. Moskva: Central'noe bjuro tehničeskoe infórmacii. 123 Seiten, Anwendung der Antibiotika in der Medizin. In: (Herausgeber) Volkswirtschaftsrat der Stadt Moskau; Reihe: Ergebnisse der Wissenschaft und Technik. Anwendung der Antibiotika in der Medizin. Gekürzte Stenogramme der Konferenz vom 24. und 25. Dezember 1957

ESTELLE, Ariana: Kombucha 1001. Harwood, Texas, USA, 76 pages

factum (df): Das Gehirn als Kopf der Abwehrkraft. factum 10/1988, 431-432

FASCHING, R.: Krebs heilen mit dem Teepilz Kombucha. Diagnosen 8 (10/1986), 62-65

FASCHING, R.: Pilz gegen Pilz. Diagnosen 8 (11/1986), 64-66

FASCHING, R.: Teepilz Kombucha, das Naturheilmittel und seine Bedeutung bei Krebs und anderen Stoffwechselkrankheiten, 72 Seiten, 10. Auflage, Ennsthaler Verlag Steyr, 1988

FISCHER, G.: Heilkräuter und Arzneipflanzen, 5. Auflage, neu bearbeitet von E. Krug, Haug, Heidelberg 1978

FISCHER, Wolfgang u. Friedrich PETERMANN: Leben ohne Sauerstoff. 116 Seiten, Urania-Verlag Leipzig, Jena, 1979

FLÜCK, V. u. E. STEINEGGER: Eine neue Hefekomponente des Teepilzes. Scientia pharmaceutica (Wien) 25 (1957), 43-44

FONTANA J.D., FRANCO V.C., DE SOUZA S.J., LYRA I.N., DE SOUZA A.M. 1991. Nature of plant stimulators in the production of Acetobacter xylinum (tea fungus) biofilm used in skin therapy. Appl. Biochem. Biotechnol. 28: 341-351

FRANK, Günther W.: Kombucha – Das Teepilzgetränk. Praxisgerechte Anleitung für die Zubereitung und Anwendung. 15th edition, 176 Seiten (German language), 2000, W. ENNSTHALER (Eds), Steyr, Austria

FRANK Günther W.: Kombucha, la boisson au champignon de longue vie. Instructions pratiques de préparation et d'utilisation. 150 pages (French language), 1990, W. ENNSTHALER (Eds), Steyr, Austria

FRANK, Günther W.: Koemboecha – De Theezwamdrank. Praktische handleiding voor toebereiding en gebruik, 150 pages (Dutch language), 1991, W. ENNSTHALER (Eds), Steyr, Austria

FRANK, Günther: Kombucha (Antwort auf eine Leseranfrage). Sonnseitig leben (Zürich) 40. Nr. 214, Juni/Juli 1989, 20

FRANK, Günther: Kombucha-Essig. Sonnseitig leben (Zürich) 41. Nr. 220, Juni/Juli 1990, 16

FRANK, Günther: Der Teepilz Kombucha. Sonnseitig leben (Zürich) 41. Nr. 219, April/Mai 1990, 16

FRANK, Günther: Der Teepilz Kombucha. Sonnseitig leben (Zürich) 41, Nr. 218 (Febr./März 1990), 17

FRANK, Günther: Der Teepilz Kombucha – ein Wundermittel? Natur & Heilen (München) 67 (4/1990), 180-186

FRANK, Günther W.: Hausmittel gegen Bresten und Gebrechen. Der Teepilz Kombucha und die Meereskristalle Tibi als Gesundheitselixiere. Natürlich (Aarau/Schweiz) 10, 11/1990, 68-72

FRANK, Günther: Gesundheitsfördernde Wirkungen des Kombucha Tees. Natur & Heilen (München) 67 (5/1990), 240-245

FRANK, Günther W.:Kombucha-Tee selbst herstellen schädlich? (Antwort auf eine Leseranfrage) Natur & Heilen (München) 68, Nr. 8/1991, August 1991), 434-435

FRANK, Günther W.:The Fascination of the Kombucha. The american raum & zeit (Mount Vernon, USA) Vol. 2 (5/1991), 51-56

FRANK, Günther W.: Die Symbiose Kombucha – Das alte, neuentdeckte Volksheilmittel zum Selbermachen. Naturheilpraxis 44, Nr. 6/91, 591-596

FRANK, Günther W.: Der Teepilz Kombucha. Amadea Nr. 3, Dezember 1991, 4-7

FRANK, Günther W.: Faszination Kombucha. Sonnseitig leben (Zürich) 42, Nr. 228 (Okt./Nov. 1991), 21-22

FRANK, Günther W.: Kombucha – das alte, neuentdeckte Volksheilmittel. Sonnseitig leben (Zürich) 42, Nr. 229 (Dez. 91/ Jan. 92), 13-14

FRANK, Günther W.: Kombucha – der Pilz des langen Lebens. Sonnseitig leben (Zürich) 43, Nr. 231 (April/Mai 1992), 3, 16, 20

FRANK, Günther: Aus dem fernen Osten. Das Alternative Branchenbuch (München), 5. Ausgabe 1992/1993, 369

FRANK, Günther W.: Kombucha's Ever Increasing Popularity. Explore more (Mt. Vernon/USA) Number 12, July/August 1995, 44-45

FRANK, Günther W.: Kombucha's Ever Increasing Popularity. Explore, (Mt. Vernon/USA) Volume 6, Number 3, June 1995, 28

FRANK, Günther W.: Wasserkefir – Geschwister des Teepilzes Kombucha. Natur & Heilen (München) 72, 6/1995, 300-305

FRANK, Günther W.: Wasserkefir – Geschwister des Teepilzes Kombucha. Natur und Medizin (Bonn) 3/95 (Mai/Juni 1995), 13-16

FRANK, Rosemarie: Die Faszination von Kombucha. 12 Seiten. Birkenfeld 1993

FRANK, H. K.: Einführung in das Mykotoxinproblem. 3-9. In: Reiß, J. (Hrsg.): Mykotoxine in Lebensmitteln. Gustav Fischer Verlag. Stuttgart 1981

FRANZ, G.: Polysaccharide mit Antitumorwirkung. Cesra-Säule 50 (1988), 7-11

FRANZ, G. u. J. KRAUS: Pflanzliche Polysaccharide mit Antitumorwirkung. Zeitschrift für Phytotherapie 8 (1987), 114

FROMMHOLZ, Jürgen: Ein asiatischer Bio-Krafttrunk verhilft zu Höchstleistungen. Bio spezial (Tutzing) Nr. 5/1991, 43

FUNKE, Hans: Der Teepilz Kombucha. Natur & Heilen 64 (1987), 509-513

GARMS, H.: Pflanzenkunde II, 8. Auflage, 183 Seiten, Westermann-Verlag, Braunschweig 1964

GEIS, Heide-Marie Karin: Ein Pilz für alle Fälle. Kraut & Rüben (München) Nr. 9/1990 (September 1990), 78-80

GEO, Heft November 1987: Grüner Tee hemmt Tumoren, Seite 174, Gruner & Jahr, Hamburg

GESELLSCHAFT für biologische Krebsabwehr e.V., Heidelberg: Merkblatt über biologische Krebsabwehr. 1984

GLAS, Gerhard: Wie wird das Kombucha-Getränk angesetzt? hp-Kurier 19 (4/1987), 89

GÖTZ, Georg: Kombucha – der Wunderpilz, der Millionen Gesundheit schenkt. 12 Folgen in "Das Neue", Hefte 3 (18.01.88) bis 14 (02.04.1988). Heinrich Bauer Verlag, Hamburg

GOLZ, Helmut: Kombucha – ein altes Teeheilmittel schenkt neue Gesundheit. 132 Seiten, Ariston Verlag Genf. ISBN 3-7205-1596-6

GROENEVELD, M. u. C. LEITZMANN: Zum Vorkommen antikanzerogener Substanzen in Lebensmitteln. Aktuelle Ernährung 12 (1987), 202-204

GÜNTER, Martin: Nachlese zum "Religionskrieg" in Küche und Kochbuch, Abschnitt Kombucha-Teepilz. Raum & Zeit (Sauerlach) 10, Nr. 57 (Mai/Juni 1992), 41-47

HAEHN, H. u. M. ENGEL: Über die Bildung von Milchsäure durch Bacterium xylinum. Milchsäuregärung durch Kombucha. Zentralblatt für Bakteriologie, Mikrobiologie und Hygiene, II. Abt. Ref. 79 (1929), 182-185

HÄNSEL, Rudolf und SCHIMMITAT, Irene: Was ist wirklich dran am Kombucha-Pilz? Ärztliche Praxis 16, Nr. 45 vom 06.06.1989, 1704-1705

HAGER, Hermann (Begr.); P. H. LIST u. L. HÖRHAMMER (Hrsg.): Hagers Handbuch der Pharmazeutischen Praxis für Apotheker, Arzneimittelhersteller und Medizinalbeamte. 4. Band, 4. Neuausgabe, Springer-Verlag, Berlin/Heidelberg/New York 1973

HAHMANN, C.: Über Drogen und Drogenverfälschungen. Apotheker-Zeitung 44 (37/1929), 561-563, S. 563

HAMM, M.: Kleine Ernährungslehre – praxisnah. Herz, Sport und Gesundheit Nr. 1/1988, 70-72

HARMS, H.: Der japanische Teepilz. Therapeutische Berichte, Leverkusen (1927), 498-500

HARNISCH, Günter: Kombucha – geballte Heilkraft aus der Natur. 1991, Turm-Verlag Bietigheim, 160 Seiten.

HALPENNY & McDERMOTT: The Effects of Tea Drinking. Canad. M. Ass. J. 41 (1939), 449

HAUSER S.P. 1990. Dr. Sklenar's kombucha mushroom infusion-a biological cancer therapy. Schweiz Rundsch. Med. Prax. 79:243-246.

HECKER, Michael u. Wolfgang BABEL: Physiologie der Mikroorganismen. 304 Seiten. Gustav Fischer Verlag, Stuttgart, New York, 1988

HEEDE, K.-O.: Millionen könnten geheilt werden. 1. Auflage, 336 Seiten, Verlag Mehr Wissen, Düsseldorf 1985

HEIMANN, W.: Grundzüge der Lebensmittelchemie, 3. Auflage, Steinkopff-Verlag, Darm-stadt 1976

HEINZELMANN, Rolf: Kombucha – eine bemerkenswerte Flechte. Obst und Garten (Stuttgart) 113, Nr. 2/1994, 40-41

HENDLER, S. S.: The complete guide to anti-aging nutrients, Seite 136, Fireside 1984

HENNEBERG, W.: Zur Kenntnis der Schnellessig- und Weinessigbakterien, Zentralblatt für Bakteriologie, Abt. II, 17 (25/1907), 789-804

HENNEBERG, W.: Handbuch der Gärungsbakteriologie, 1. Band (Allgemeine Gärungsbakte-

riologie, Praktikum und Betriebsuntersuchungen. Unter besonderer Berücksichtigung der Hefe-, Essig- und Milchsäurepilze), 2. Auflage, 604 Seiten, Verlag Paul Parey, Berlin 1926 (a)

HENNEBERG, W.: Handbuch der Gärungsbakteriologie, 2. Band (Spezielle Pilzkunde, unter besonderer Berücksichtigung der Hefe-, Essig- und Milchsäurebakterien), 2. Auflage, 404 Seiten, Verlag Paul Parey, Berlin 1926 (b)

HENRY, Linda: Kombucha – Bodybuilding's wonder mushroom. Muscle and Fitness, June 1995, pages 178 -184

HERMANN, S.: Über die sogenannte Kombucha, I. Biochemische Zeitschrift 192 (1928), 176-199

HERMANN, S.: Über die sogenannte Kombucha, II. Biochemische Zeitschrift 192 (1928), 188-199

HERMANN, S.: Die sogenannte "Kombucha". Umschau 33 (1929), 841-844

HERMANN, S. u. N. FODOR: C-Vitamin-(l-Ascorbinsäure)-Bildung durch eine Symbiose von Essigbakterien und Hefen. Biochemische Z. 276 (5-6/1935), 323-325

HEROLD, Edmund: Heilwerte aus dem Bienenvolk. Ehrenwirth Verlag, München

HESSELTINE, C. W.: A Millenium of fungi, food, and fermentation. Mycologia 57 (New York). (1965), 149-197

HOBBS, Christopher: Kombucha, Manchurian Tea Mushroom, Thew Essential Guide. 57 pages. Santa Cruz, California, 1995

HOBBYTHEK: Rund um den Tee. 1987, 14-17

HOBBY-TIP der HOBBYTHEK, Nr. 134: "Herzhaft und gesund" (1986)

HOFFMANN, Norbert: The Rest of the Story. 2000. The information provided here focuses primarily on the more scientific aspects of the Kombucha culture. Some is based on Hoffmann's own lab tests and literature research, some may be excerpts from documents Norbert Hoffmann has discovered or received from others.

OUR BLUE MARBLE: http://www.ourbluemarble.us/norbert/kombucha/

IRION, H. (Hrsg.): Fungus japonicus, Fungojapon Kombucha – Indisch-japanischer Teepilz. In: Lehrgang für Drogistenfachschulen in 4 Bänden, Band 2: Botanik/Drogenkunde. 4. Auflage, S. 405, 528 Seiten, Verlagsgesellschaft Rudolf Müller, Eberswalde-Berlin-Leipzig 1944

KAMINSKI, Anette: Ärzte: Pilz heilt Frauenleiden. Bild der Frau Nr. 2 (11.01.1988). Axel Springer Verlag, Hamburg

KAŠEVNIK, L. L.: Biohimija Vitamina C. Soobščenie III. O sposobnosti japonskogo cajnogo griba sintezirovat' Vitamin C. – Bjull. exp. Biol. i Med (Moskva) 3 (1/1937), 87-88. (Die Biochemie des Vitamins C. III. Mitteilung: Die Fähigkeit des japanischen Teepilzes, Vitamin C aufzubauen). Referat: SCHWAIBOLD, N. in Chem. Zbl. 1937, II, 2860

KAŠEVNIK, L. D.: O Nekotoryh biohimiceskih osobennostjah t. n."cajnogo griba". – Sbornik trudov Archangel'skij gosudarstvennyj mediciniskij Inst. 5, 116-121. (Von einigen biochemischen Besonderheiten des sog. Teepilzes). 1940

KAŠEVNIK, L. D., PJUMINA, V. I., i NEBOLJUBOVA G. E.: Materialy k biohimii tak naz. "cajnogo griba". Soobščenie IV. O bakteriostaticeskom dejstvii èkstrakta iz nastoja "cajnogo griba". Trudy Tomskogo medicinskogo Instituta 13, 115-117. (Beiträge zur Biochemie des sog. "Teepilzes". Mitteilung IV. Über die bakteriostatischen Kräfte des Extraktes vom Aufguß des "Teepilzes".) 1946

KAUFMANN, Klaus: Kombucha Rediscovered! 82 pages, Burnaby BC Canada, 1995

KIEFER, T.: Va et vient: Kombucha. Televion broadcast on May 08, 1996. TF 1 (French television station "France 1")

KLETTER, Christa: Kombucha – der Teepilz. Deutsche Apotheker Zeitung (Stuttgart) 130, Nr. 41 vom 11.10.1990, 2266-2270

KNIERIEMEN, Heinz und Hans BERNER: Kombucha – Pilz, Flechte oder Symbiose? Natürlich (Aarau/Schweiz) 12, Nr. 6/1992, 75

KOBERT, R.: Teekwaß. Mikrokosmos 11 (1917/18), 159

KOCH, F. W.: Die Lösung des Krebsproblems durch die Anti-Acid-Methode. Anti-Acid-Nach-richten Nr. 25 und 26/1962 und Nr. 28/29/1963

KÖHLER, Valentin: Glukuronsäure macht Krebspatienten Mut. Ärztliche Praxis 33 (1981), 887

KÖHLER, V. u. J. KÖHLER: Glucuronsäure als ökologische Hilfe, S. 56-62. In: KAEGEL-MANN, H. (Hrsg. u. Mitautor): Sofortheilung des Waldes, 1. Band, 2. erweiterte Auflage, Verlag zur heilen Welt, Windecke-Rosbach 1985

KOLKWITZ, R.: Pflanzenphysiologie. 3. Auflage, Jena 1935, 113-116

KONOVALOV, I. N. u. M. A. LITVINOV u. L. M. ZAKMAN: Izmenenie prirody i fiziologi-ceskih osobennostej cajnogo griba (Medusomyces gisevii Lindau) v zavisimosti ot uslovij kul'tivi-rovanija. – Bot. zurnal (Moskava) 44 (3/1959), 346-349. (Die Veränderungen der Natur und der physiologischen Eigenschaften des Teepilzes (Medusomyces gisevii Lindau) in Beziehung zu den Bedingungen des Kulturmilieus)

KÖRNER, Helmut: Ein Parasit im Blut – Krebs. Raum & Zeit, Heft Nr. 19 (1985)

KÖRNER, Helmut: Die Heilkraft des Pilzes Kombucha. Raum & Zeit Heft 20 (Febr. 1986)

KÖRNER, Helmut: Kombucha – wertvolles Geschenk der Natur. Naturheilpraxis 39 (10/1986)

KÖRNER, Helmut: Der Teepilz Kombucha. Der Naturarzt 108 (5/1987), 14-16

KÖRNER: Helmut: Kombucha-Zubereitung wurde von Sportmedizinern getestet. Natura-med (Neckarsulm) 4 (10/1989), 592

KÖRNER, Helmut: Kombucha. Natur, Umwelt & Medizin (Heidelberg) 6, Nr. 1, Februar 1990, 40-41

KÖRNER, Helmut: Kombucha ist Immunstärker und Energiespender. Natur & Heilen (München) 68, 4/1991, 202-204

KÖRNER, Helmut: Wichtige Forschungsergebnisse mit Polysacchariden. SANUM-Post (Hoya) Nr. 28. September 1994, S. 21-22

KOZAKI, M. u. A. KOIZUMI u. K. KITAGARA: Microorganism of Zoogleal Mats Formed on Tea Decotion. J. Food Hyg. Soc. Japan 13 (1972), 89-96

KRAFT, M.-M.: Le Champignon de Thé. Nova Hedwigia 1 (3, 4/1959), 297-304

KRAUS, J. u. M. SCHNEIDER u. G. FRANZ: Antitumor polysaccharide aus Solidagosp. Deutsche Apotheker-Zeitung 126 (1986), 2045

KRAUS, Peter: Kombucha-Geschenk (Leserzuschrift). Natur & Heilen 8/1990, S. 392

KREMPL-LAMPRECHT, Luise: Aktuelle Fragen und Antworten. Pilzdialog (München) Nr. 3/1990 (August 1990), 38

KÜHNEMANN, A.-K.: Die Sprechstunde – Nachgefragt: Kombucha. Television broadcast on August, 09, 1994. (German television station "Bayern 3").

KUHL, J.: Schach dem Krebs. Humata-Verlag Harold S. Blume, Bern

LAKOWITZ, N.: Teepilz und Teekwaß. Apotheker-Zeitung 43 (1928), 298-300

LAPUZ M.M., GALARDO E.G., PALO M.A. 1967. The nata organism -cultural requirements, characerics and identity. The Philippines J. Science. 96(2): 91-109.

LESKOV, A. I.: Novye svedenija o cajnom gribe. – Fel'dser i Akuserka (Moskva) 23 (10/1958), 47-48 (Neue Angaben über den Teepilz)

LINDAU, G.: Über Medusomyces Gisevii, eine neue Gattung und Art der Hefepilze. Ber. dt. bot. Ges. 31 (1913), 243-248

LINDER, H.: Biologie. 16. Auflage, 352 Seiten, J. B. Metzlersche Verlagsbuchhandlung, Stuttgart 1967

LINDNER, P.: Über Teekwaß und Teekwaßpilze. Mikrokosmos 11 (1917), 93-98

LINDNER, P.: Die vermeintliche neue Hefe Medusomyces Gisevii. Ber. dt. bot. Ges. 31 (1913), 364-368

LIST, P. H. u. W. HUFSCHMIDT: Basische Pilzinhaltsstoffe. 5. Mitteilung über biogene Amine und Aminosäuren des Teepilzes. Pharm. Zentralhalle 98 (1959), 593-598

LÖWENHEIM, H.: Über den indischen Teepilz. Apotheker-Zeitung 42 (1927), 148-149

LÜCK, Erich: Konservierungsstoffe in Lebensmitteln – nützlich oder schädlich? Deutsche Apotheker-Zeitung 128 (1988), 510-516

MADAUS. In: Biolog. Heilkunst Nr. 15 und 20/27 (1927). Zitiert von Arauner (1929), nähere Angaben nicht zu ermitteln

MALMGREN, Berndt: Einführung in die Mikrobiologie. Aus dem Schwedischen von Solwieg Schmeller. 220 Seiten. F. K. Schattauer Verlag, Stuttgart, New York, 1976

MANN, Ulrike: Verblüffend – ein Pilz kuriert den Darm. Bild und Funk Nr. 35 (26.08.1988). Burda GmbH Offenburg

MEHNERT, H. u. H. FÖRSTER: Stoffwechselkrankheiten, 1. Auflage, 355 Seiten , Georg Thieme Verlag Stuttgart 1975

MEIXNER, A.: Combucha, der Teepilz. Südwestdeutsche Pilz-Rundschau Nr. 2/1983, 1-4

MICHL, Wendula: Herstellung von Kombucha-Tee (Leserbrief). Natur & Heilen 7/90, 340

MINDEN, Diana: Kombucha – Health Drink of the ages. 41 pages. Klamath Falls, OR/USA, 1996

MITRA, K.-K.: Tea Today, Tea Research Institute, China, nach KTM 36 (14), 15-16, o. J.

MOLLENDA, L.: Kombucha, ihre Heilbedeutung und Züchtung. Deutsche Essigindustrie 32 (27/1928), 243-244

MORELL, F.: Wasser, Bio-Elektronik Vincent. Success Express, 8 Seiten, Mai 1984

MORELL, F. u. E. RASCHE: Wasser, Lebensmittel Nr. 1. Friesenheim 1986

MORELL, F.: Wasser – Ernährung – Bioelektronik nach der Methode Vincent. Erfahrungsheilkunde 37 (10/1988), 646-651

NAUMOVA, E. K.: Meduzin – Novoe antibioticeskoe vešcestvo, obrazumoe Medusomyces Gisevi. In: Vtoraja naucnaja Konferencija sanitarnogigieniceskogo fakul'teta. 28-29 Aprelja 1949. Avtoreferaty. p. 20-23. Kazan': Kazanskij gosudarstvennyj medicinskij Institut. 55 p. (Meduzin – ein neuer antibiotischer Stoff, gebildet von Medusomyces Gisevi. In: Zweite wissenschaftliche Konferenz der Fakultät für Gesundheit und Hygiene, 28. bis 29. April 1949. Autoreferate, p. 20-23. Kazan: Kazan'sches Staatliches Medizinisches Institut. 55 p.), 1949

OETINGER-PAPENDORF, Ingeborg: Durch Entsäuerung zu seelischer und körperlicher Gesundheit. Eigenverlag, Öhringen-Ohrnberg 5, 1988

ORTH, R.: Einfluß physikalischer Faktoren auf die Bildung von Mykotoxinen. S. 85-100. In: Reiß, J. (Hrsg.): Mykotoxine in Lebensmitteln. Gustav Fischer Verlag, Stuttgart 1981

PAULA GOMES, A. de: Obsevacões sobre a utilizacão de Zymomonas mobilis (Lindner) Kluy-ver et van Niel, 1936. (Thermobacterium mobile, Lindner 1928; Pseudomonas linderi Kluyver et Hoppenbrouwers, 1931), na Térapeutica Humana. – Revista Instituto de Antibióticos (Pernambuco, Brasilien) 2 (1959), 77-81

PASCAL, Alana and Lynne Van der Kar: Kombucha – How-To and What It's All About. 128 pages. Malibu, California/USA, 1995

POPIEL, L. v.: Zur Selbstherstellung von Essig. Pharmaz. Post (Wien) 50 (80/1917), 757-758

POSTGATE, John: Mikroben, unsere Freunde – unsere Feinde. 184 Seiten, Umschau Verlag, Frankfurt, 1970

PRO 7 (German television station) on August 24, 1995: Kombucha (a report on Günther W. Frank)

PRYOR, B. und Sanford Holst: Kombucha Phenomen. The health drink sweeping America. 120 pages, Sherman Oaks, California, 1995

PRYOR, B.: The Kombucha Tea Mushroom and AIDS. Whole Life Times (Malibu, CA), May 1994, 14-15, 46

PLETZNITZKY, A., Ars Medici (Wien) 17 (1927), 604

PSCHYREMBEL, W. (Begr.); C. ZINK (Bearb.): Pschyrembel Klinisches Wörterbuch, 255. Auflage, 1873 Seiten, de Gruyter, Berlin/New York, 1986

PUNSAR, S. und Mitarbeiter: Coronary heart disease and drinking water. J. Chron. Dis. 28 (1975), 259-287

PÜTZ, J.: Das Hobbythek-Buch, Band 3, 5. Auflage, Verlagsgesellschaft Schulfernsehen, Köln 1984

REICHHOLF-RIEHM, H.: Insekten, 287 Seiten, Mosaik Verlag, München 1983

REISS, Jürgen: Der Teepilz und seine Stoffwechselprodukte. Deutsche Lebensmittel-Rundschau 83 (9/1987), 286-290

REISS J. 1989. Influence of different sugars on the metabolism of the tea. Z. Lebensm. Unters. Forsch. 198:258-261.

REITZ, M. u. P. GUTJAHR: Krebs, was ist das? 405 Seiten, Ullstein, Frankfurt 1983

Rick, Marin und N.A. Biddle: Trends: Taking the Fungal-Tea Plunge. Newsweek Vol. LXXV, No. 2, 9. Januar 1995, Seite 64, New York.

ROUJON, L.: Theorie und Praxis der Bio-Elektronik Vincent. SIBEV-Verlag, Wenden-Ottfin-gen, 1975

ROOTS, H.: Teeseeneleotise Ravitoimest. Noukogude eesti tervishoid (Talin, Estland) (2/1959), 55-57 (Die Heilkräfte des Teepilzes)

ROSS P., MAYER ., BENZIMAN M. 1991. Cellulose biosynthesis and function in bacteria. Microbiological Reviews. 44:35-58.

RÜCKERT, Ulrich: Wunderheiler Kombucha-Pilz. Frau im Spiegel Nr. 28 vom 01. Juli 1998, Seiten 66-67. Verlag Ehrlich & Sohn GmbH & Co., Postfach 50 04 45, 22704 Hamburg

S.: Der "japanische Teepilz" – Die Weiße Fahne, Zeitblätter zur Verinnerlichung und Vergeistigung (Pfullingen, Württemberg) 9 (4/1928), 184-185

SACHSSE, Joachim: Vorbeugen gegen Krebs durch biologische Früherkennungsmethoden, 2. Auflage, 108 Seiten, Verlag Mehr Wissen, Düsseldorf 1984

ŠAKARJAN, G. A. u. L. T. DANIELOVA: Antibiotičeskie svojstva nastoja griba Medusomyces gisevii (čajnogo griba). Soobščenie 1. – Trudy Erevanskogo zooveterinarnogo Instituta, 10 (1948), 33-45. (Die antibiotischen Fähigkeiten des Aufgusses von Medusomyces gisevii (Teepilz) 1. Mitteilung)

SANDER, F.: Der Säure-Basen-Haushalt des menschlichen Organismus. Hippokrates-Verlag, Stuttgart 1953

SCHAERTEL, M.: Ober, ein Pilz bitte (a report on Günther W. Frank). FOCUS (Munich) No. 34, August 21, 1995, page 128

SCHLEGEL, Hans G. unter Mitarbeit von Karin SCHMIDT: Allgemeine Mikrobiologie. 6. überarbeitete Auflage, 571 Seiten, Georg Thieme Verlag, Stuttgart, New York, 1985

SCHMIDT, Ingrid: Der Teepilz – morphologische, physiologische und therapeutische Untersu-chungen. 51 Seiten, Schriftliche Hausarbeit im Rahmen der Ersten Staatsprüfung für das Lehramt Sekundarstufe I., Bochum 1979

SCHNEIDRZIK, W. E. J.: Die richtige Arznei, 352 Seiten, Gustav Lübbe Verlag, Bergisch Gladbach, 1985

SCHNITZER, J. G.: Der alternative Weg zur Gesundheit. Schnitzer, St. Georgen 1982

SCHMEIL, O. u. A. SEYBOLD: Lehrbuch der Botanik, 1. Band, 50. Auflage, 400 Seiten, Ver-lag von Quelle und Meyer, Leipzig 1940

SCHMEIL, O. u. A. SEYBOLD: Lehrbuch der Botanik, 2. Band, 50. Auflage, 303 Seiten, Ver-lag von Quelle und Meyer, Leipzig 1941

SCHÖN, Georg: Mikrobiologie. 144 Seiten, Verlag Herder, Freiburg 1978

SCHRÖDER, Helga: Mikrobiologisches Praktikum. 220 Seiten, Volk und Wissen, Volkseigener Verlag, Berlin 1975

SCHUITEMAKER, G.E.: Immunkrankheiten. ORTHOsupplement (Baarn, Netherlands) Nr. 1, 1988, 1-3

SCHULTZ-FRIESE, W. u. G. GADAL: Rezepte für eine krebsfeindliche Vollwertkost. Bir-cher Benner Verlag, Bad Homburg 1980

SCHULZ, K. H.: Psychoneuroimmunologie. Zeitschrift für Allgemeinmedizin 62 (26/1986), 871-878

SCHWAIBOLD, N.: Referat über: KAŠEVNIK, L. D., 1937, Chem. Zbl. 1937, II. 2860

SEEGER, G. P.: Das Krebsproblem unter dem Blickfeld des Milchsäurestoffwechsels und die Bedeutung der Milchsäure als Vorbeugungmittel, Heilkunde und Heilwege, Heft 4/1952

SEEGER, P. G. u. J. SACHSSE: Krebsverhütung durch biologische Vorsorgemaßnahmen. 148 Seiten, Verlag Mehr Wissen, Düsseldorf 1984

SESHADRI, R., S. NAGALAKSHMI, J. MADHUSUDHANA RAO und C.P. NATARAJAN: Utilization of by-products of the tea plant: a review. Tropical Agriculture (Trinidad) 63, Nr. 1, Januar 1986, 2-6

SKLENAR, Rudolf: Ein in der Iris sichtbarer Test für eine Stoffwechselstörung, kontrolliert an Hand von Dunkelfelduntersuchungen des Blutes nach Scheller. Erfahrungsheilkunde 13 (3/1964).

SKLENAR, Rudolf: Krebsdiagnose aus dem Blut und die Behandlung von Krebs, Präkanzero-sen und sonstigen Stoffwechselkrankheiten mit der Kombucha und Colipräparaten. 8 Seiten, o. J.

SOURNIA, J. C. und Mitarbeiter: Illustrierte Geschichte der Medizin in 9 Bänden, Band 1, Ver-lag Andreas & Andreas, Salzburg 1980 (S. 79-81)

SOURNIA, J. C. und Mitarbeiter: Illustrierte Geschichte der Medizin in 9 Bänden, Band 2, Verlag Andreas & Andreas, Salzburg 1980 S. 655-656 (Kapitel "Die japanische Medizin" von Alain Briot) : "In der Tat verfügte Japan erst etwa im vierten Jahrhundert unserer Zeitrechnung über eine elaborierte Medizin. Da es bis zu dieser Zeit kein Schriftsystem besaß, nahm es – mit mehr oder weniger Glück – die chinesische Schrift an. Gewöhnlich datieren wir die offizielle Einführung der kontinentalen Medizin auf das Jahr 414 unserer Zeitrechnung, als nämlich der koreanische Mediziner Kombu aus dem Königreich Sylla mit dem Auftrag in Japan eintraf, den Kaiser Inkyo zu behandeln."

STADELMANN, Eduard: Der Teepilz. Eine Literaturzusammenstellung. Sydowia, Ann. myco-log. Ser. II., 11 (1957), 380-388

STADELMANN, Eduard: Der Teepilz und seine antibiotische Wirkung (Eine Bibliographie). Zentralblatt Bakt. I. Abt. Ref. 180 (1961), 401-435

STADELMANN, Eduard https://web.archive.org/web/20100217052230/ http://horticulture.cfans.umn.edu/sites/89c81b82-b540-417a-96b4-5b46174c-cd79/uploads/kombucha.htm

STAMETS, Paul: My Adventures with the Blob. Mushroom the Journal, Winter 1994-95, page 5 – 9,

STEIGER, K. E. u. E. STEINEGGER: Über den Teepilz. Pharmaceutica Acta Helvetiae 32 (1957), 133-154

STEPP, W. u. J. KÜHNAU u. H. SCHRÖDER: Die Vitamine und ihre klinische Anwendung. 6. Auflage, Ferdinand Enke Verlag, Stuttgart 1944

STRAUSS, E.: Zur Anwendung der Milchsäure in der Behandlung Malignomkranker. Deut-sches Gesundheitswesen, DDR, Heft 27/1977

SUKIASJAN, A. O.: Vlijanie faktorov vnešnej sredy i istocnikov pitanija na nakoplenie antiblo-tlceskih veščestv v kul'ture "cajnogo griba". Soobščenie I. Izucenie razlicnyh fiziko-mehaniceskih vozodejstvij. – Trudy Erevanskogo zooveterinarnogo Instituta 17, 229-235, 1954; (Der Einfluß von Milieufaktoren und Nährstoffquellen auf die Anreicherung von antibiotischen Stoffen in den Kulturen des Teepilzes. I. Mitteilung. Untersuchung verschiedener physikomechanischer Einflüsse)

SÜSSMUTH, Roland, J. EBERSPÄCHER, R. HAAG u. W. SPRINGER: Biochemischmikrobiologisches Praktikum. 409 Seiten, Georg Thieme Verlag, Stuttgart, New York, 1987

TIETZE, Harald: Kombucha. The miracle fungus. 112 pages, Bath/Uk 1995

TIMMONS, Stuart: Fungus among us. New Age Journal Volume XI, Issue 7, November/December 1994, pages 78 – 81 and 88 – 96 (New Age Publishing Inc., Watertown, MA 02172

TROLL, W.: Allgemeine Botanik. 4. Auflage, Ferdinand Enke Verlag, Stuttgart 1973

TSCHIRCH, A.: Handbuch der Pharmakognosie. 2. Band, Tauchnitz, Leipzig 1912 (s. 306)

UHLENBRUCK, G.: Neuropeptide – Dirigenten des Immunorchesters. Ärztliche Praxis 40 (105/1988), 3263

UTKIN, L.: o novom mikroorganizme iz gruppy uksusnyh bakterij. – Mikrobiologia (Moskva) 6 (4/1937), 421-434. (Über einen neuen Mikroorganismus aus der Gruppe der Essigsäurebakterien). Referat: GORDIENKO, M., Zbl. Bakt. 98 (1937), II. 359.

VALENTIN, H.: Über die Verwendung des indischen Teepilzes und seine Gewinnung in trockener Form. Apotheker-Zeitung 43 (1928), 1533-1536

VALENTIN, H.: Wesenliche Bestandteile der Gärungsprodukte in den durch Pilztätigkeit gewonnenen Hausgetränken sowie die Verbreitung der letzteren. Apotheker-Zeitung 45 (1930), 1464-1465 und 1477-1478

VALENTINE, Tom: Kombucha -Ancient ferment with a healthy promise. Search for Health vo. 1, number 6, July/August 1993, pages 2 – 14

VALENTINE, Tom: Kombucha; A Traditional Fermented Drink Sweeps America. in: Search for Health – A Classic Anthology, Pages 426 – 448, Naples, Florida 1996

VALENTINE, Tom: Kombucha Update. Search for Health Vol. 3, No. 2+3, Nov. 94/February 1995, pages 25 to 37

VOGEL, A.: Der kleine Doktor. 33. Auflage, 861 Seiten, Verlag A. Vogel, Teufen (Schweiz) 1977

VOGEL, A.: Krebs. 405 Seiten, Verlag A. Vogel, Teufen (Schweiz) 1987

VOGEL, A.: Krebs-Früherkennung. Gesundheits-Nachrichten 6/1988, S. 88-89

WALDECK, H.: Der Teepilz. Pharmazeutische Zentralhalle 68 (1927), 789-790

WEIDE, Heinz u. Harald AURICH: Allgemeine Mikrobiologie. 519 Seiten, Gustav Fischer Verlag, Stuttgart, New York, 1979

WEIDINGER, Hermann-Josef: Kombucha, "Tee" der aus dem Meere kam. Ringelblume Nr. 4/ 1988, 25-33

WEINSTOCK, D.: Pflanzliches in der Krebstherapie, Südwestpresse (Ulm), 12.01.1987

WELZL, E.: Biochemie der Ernährung. De Gruyter, Berlin 1985

WERNER: Polysaccharide als Immunstimmulanzien. Deutsche Apotheker-Zeitung 128 (21/ 1988), 1127-1128

Westdeutscher Rundfunk, 15.06.98, 18:20 bis 18:50: Service-Zeit, Kostprobe: "Kombucha – Wundertee mit viel Geschmack" von Fromut Pott (siehe auch http:// www.wdr.de/tv/kostprobe/kp_sarchiv/1998/06/15_3.html)

WIECHOWSKI, W.: Welche Stellung soll der Arzt zur Kombuchafrage einnehmen? Beiträge zur ärztlichen Fortbildung 6 (1/1928), 2-10

WILLIAMS W.S., CANNON R.E. 1989. Alternative environmental roles for cellulose produced by Acetobacter xylinum. Appl. Env. Microbiol. 55:2248-2252.

WILKINSON, John Frederick: Einführung in die Mikrobiologie. Aus dem Englischen von Barbara Schröder. 162 Seiten. Verlag Chemie, Weinheim, 1974

WOLLER, R.: Häufigkeit des Vorkommens von Mykotoxinen in der Bundesrepublik Deutschland. S. 143-170. In: Reiß, J. (Hrsg.): Mykotoxine in Lebensmitteln. Gustav Fischer Verlag, Stuttgart 1981

ZETTKIN-SCHALDACH, (Hrsg.) von Heinz DAVID: Wörterbuch der Medizin, Zahnheilkunde und Grenzgebiete. 2 Bände, 7. neubearb. und erw. Auflage, 2345 Seiten, Georg Thieme Verlag, Stuttgart 1985

Zydeck, Franziska: Kombucha – Pilz mit Power. Bolero (Zürich) Nr. 1/2 Januar/Februar 1997, 82-83

About the Author

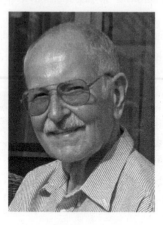

Günther W. Frank lives in Birkenfeld in the Black Forest, is married and has four children. He is deeply passionate about microbiology and naturopathy.

The graduate in public administration wanted to get to the bottom of the ancient legend surrounding the kombucha mushroom and for years he has been driven by the notion of finding the truth behind it. He has not been able to get the kombucha mushroom, this small chemical factory which produces various organic acids and other substances out of his mind. Günther W. Frank has gone from being a huge skeptic to an absolutely convinced supporter of the tea mushroom beverage. His book is known as the best "Kombucha Bible" not only in Europe, but also in many other countries.